WORKING WITH DREAMS
IN PSYCHOTHERAPY

THE PRACTICING PROFESSIONAL
A Guilford Series

Edited by

MICHAEL J. MAHONEY

SELF-NARRATIVES: THE CONSTRUCTION
OF MEANING IN PSYCHOTHERAPY
Herbert J. M. Hermans and Els Hermans-Jansen

FOCUSING-ORIENTED PSYCHOTHERAPY:
A MANUAL OF THE EXPERIENTIAL METHOD
Eugene T. Gendlin

WORKING WITH DREAMS IN PSYCHOTHERAPY
Clara E. Hill

Working with Dreams in Psychotherapy

Clara E. Hill

THE GUILFORD PRESS
New York   London

© 1996 The Guilford Press
A Division of Guilford Publications, Inc.
72 Spring Street, New York, NY 10012

Library of Congress Cataloging-in-Publication Data

Hill, Clara E.
    Working with dreams in psychotherapy / Clara E. Hill.
        p.   cm. — (The practicing professional)
    Includes bibliographical references and index.
    ISBN 1-57230-092-2
    1. Dream interpretation. 2. Psychoanalytic interpretation.
3. Psychotherapy.   I. Title. II. Series.
    [DNLM: 1. Dreams—psychology. 2. Psychoanalytic Interpretation.
2. Psychotherapy—methods. WM 460.5.D8 H645w 1996]
RC489.D74H55 1996
616.89′14—dc20
DNLM/DLC
for Library of Congress   96-14095
                                                                      CIP

Preface

I BECAME INTERESTED IN dream interpretation when I taught an undergraduate course in theories of personality and a graduate course in theories and strategies of counseling and psychotherapy. When presenting the theories of Freud, Jung, Adler, and Perls, I demonstrated their methods of dream interpretation with students in the class who volunteered to tell a dream. Of course, I emphasized to the students that we were "playing" and demonstrating the approach rather than doing therapy. I further indicated to the students telling the dreams that they could stop at any point they wished. I vividly remember one of the first students for the Freudian dream interpretation naively presenting a dream about wanting a hot dog—needless to say, the class roared.

Both undergraduate and graduate students loved the classes on dream interpretation. Their questions about dreams and their disclosures about the effects of their dreams on them in their waking lives convinced me that dreams are highly meaningful and important. Students came back years later and told me they still thought about the dreams that we interpreted in class.

So, when I had the opportunity to teach a special seminar, I decided to delve further into dreams. In the first seminar with undergraduate honors students, I focused on the variety of different theories of dream interpretation. I was most attracted to the Freudian, Jungian, and Gestalt methods of dream interpretation and attended several workshops to learn more about these approaches.

One of the exciting things about teaching is that students challenge your ideas. In this case, the students from the experimental areas of psychology challenged the clinical theories about dreams. To refute these ideas, I began reading more about the physiology and cognitive bases of dreaming. Unfortunately, the empirical research did not seem to support the psychodynamic approaches to dream interpretation that I was advocating. There was no evidence that dreams were a "message from the unconscious," that dreams represented wish fulfillments, or that symbols in dreams had any fixed meaning. If dreams are just random bursts of brain activity (Hobson & McCarley, 1977), the brain purging itself of irrelevant information that accumulates during the day (Crick & Mitchison, 1983), or simply information processing (Palombo, 1978, 1980, 1987), who really cares about them? Much as I may have wanted to, I could not summarily dismiss these hypotheses about the lack of psychological significance in the formation of dreams, because they made some sense.

On the other hand, the clinical theories about dreams also made sense. Freud and Jung and other psychologists whom I respected could not be totally wrong about the value of dream interpretation in therapy. Furthermore, dream interpretation seemed to work: my students had profited from it, my clients in therapy seemed to benefit from working with their dreams, and I had found it valuable when I remembered and discussed my own dreams with my therapist. There seemed to be something to dream interpretation regardless of where dreams came from or what they meant.

Being a good scientist, I went to the literature. But there was no empirical research on dream interpretation. Fortunately, I had students who were excited about dream interpretation, so we embarked on a series of studies to determine the efficacy of dream interpretation (see Chapter 12). Along the way, I had to develop a model of dream interpretation so that we would have a standard method for the therapists we trained. I discovered that I had definite ideas about what seemed to work in dream interpretation. As we trained therapists for our studies, thought about the results of our research, and integrated the research on sleep, dreaming, and cognition, I developed and refined the approach presented in this book. The model has gone through many revisions, and I expect that it will go through many more.

My hope is that the model I have presented is flexible enough to be used by many types of therapists. It is a model that stresses learning about the dream from the client's perspective through extensive *exploration,* then putting together the exploration into some coherent *interpretation,* and then attending to the message of the dream by helping the client take some *action* and make changes.

At this point, I firmly believe in the value of dream interpretation, particularly for those people who recall their dreams, are motivated to work with their dreams, and are insight oriented. I am excited about the preliminary results of our research and hope that there will be much more research to determine the effective components of dream interpretation.

I want to acknowledge and thank the wonderful students I have had over the years who helped me develop and test this dream interpretation model. In particular, Susan Brandt, Mary Cogar, Roberta Diemer, Dana Falk, Kristin Heaton, Shirley Hess, Anne Hillyer, Annie

Judge, Sarah Knox, Leslie Lobell, Beth Pontari, David Peterson, Anne Regan, Peggy Rios, Aaron Rochlen, Robyn Seeman, Barbara Vivino, and Jason Zack have talked with me endlessly about this model, used it in sessions with clients, and/or read numerous drafts of this book. In addition, I want to thank Anne Sachs and Wendy Kurtz for typing transcripts of dream interpretation sessions and Dorothy Bradford for checking references. I also want to thank several colleagues, Nancy Anderson, Jim Gormally, Barbara Thompson, and Renee Rhodes, who read various parts and drafts of the book and provided helpful feedback. A theory develops out of extended discussion with students and colleagues who are willing to share and challenge ideas, so I am grateful to these folks for the dialogue. In addition, I presented portions of this book in my Presidential Address at the Society for Psychotherapy Research in Vancouver, British Columbia, Canada, on June 22, 1995 (the text of that talk is published in Hill, 1996). Finally, I want to thank my therapist, Rona Eisner, who taught me much through working with me on my own dreams in therapy.

I hope that you too will become excited about dreams and dream interpretation as you read through this book and begin to work with dreams.

Contents

PART I

Background

CHAPTER ONE

The Role of Dream Interpretation

I see a skeleton mounted on and riding a white horse. The horse has red glowing eyes. I am then in what appears to be a graveyard with my children. The horse has trampled over my ex-husband, and he appears to be dead. The sun is rising and has risen completely before the end of the dream. All is silent except for the river that flows not far away. As the sun rises, birds begin to chirp, and one can even hear fish jumping in the river. The skeleton continues on quietly on the horse, and one can't even hear the horse's hooves.

I am underwater on a mechanical device that rides up and down. The water is murky. I am observing ocean floor creatures all coated with this deep water sediment. Everything is monochrome. I move up, riding on the machine, and the platform I am on is level with the water. Something is on my back. It is an octopus and it sticks to my back. I try to get it off, but new parts keep sticking. Finally, I tear it off and throw it in the water.

THESE DREAMS, reported as a part of our study on dream groups for recently separated and divorcing women (Falk & Hill, 1995), illustrate how vivid, salient, and frightening dreams can be. They also illustrate how waking issues are incorporated into dreams and that dreams represent an attempt to process emotional issues, in this case the experience of divorce.

Clients often present vivid and troubling dreams like these in therapy. Such dreams can leave clients feeling so frightened and anxious that they wake up and cannot return to sleep. They wonder what these dreams mean. Some clients ruminate about their dreams, wondering if doing things in dreams (e.g., killing their parents, having sex with their child) means that they have the capacity to act out these behaviors in waking life.

Some clients, particularly those suffering from posttraumatic stress disorder (PTSD), have nightmares in which they repeatedly reexperience a traumatic event, such as a rape or murder. Others have recurrent dreams that are not exact replays of a specific traumatic event but repeat a traumatic theme in a metaphorical manner. Examples of typical recurrent dreams are dreams of being chased or flunking a class. These recurrent dreams or nightmares seem to reflect ongoing problems that the person has not resolved (Cartwright & Lamberg, 1992).

WHY THERAPISTS
DO NOT EXAMINE DREAMS IN THERAPY

Unfortunately, therapists often dismiss dreams as being "just dreams," rather than fully exploring them to help their clients understand and integrate the meanings. These therapists miss an excellent therapeutic opportunity because dreams reflect waking life in a way that often affects people at a deep, metaphorical level. Any event from waking life that was as vivid, salient, and troubling as some dreams can be would undoubtedly be explored in therapy. Why not dreams? Indeed, we spend about 2 hours a night in the dreaming state, so dreams constitute a large part of our existence and should be a focus of therapy when clients are troubled by them.

Some therapists recognize the importance of dreams but fail to explore them adequately because they lack the training or knowledge about how to integrate dreamwork into ongoing therapy. Others believe that dreams are either trivial, meaningless, impossible to decipher, nonscientific, or associated with the occult. Weiss (1986) proposed that relatively few therapists use dream analysis in their work because of the many misconceptions associated with it. For example, many feel that dream interpretation is used only by psychoanalysts and that dream interpretation takes people away from waking concerns into obscure meanderings in the unconscious. Similarly, some therapists think of dream interpretation as something that occurs only in long-term therapy because it takes so long to uncover all the disguised latent content.

BENEFITS OF WORKING
WITH DREAMS IN THERAPY

Dream interpretation can play an important role in long-term therapy. With the luxury of unlimited time, therapists and clients can explore the depths of the client's personality through dreams. Themes can be derived from series of dreams, and changes in dream content over the course of therapy can be charted.

Dream interpretation also, however, has an important place in brief therapy. Dream interpretation often leads directly to a person's central conflicts even though the person previously could not articulate what was making him or her unhappy. Often clients are out of touch with what is truly troubling them, but quickly become aware of troubling issues when they associate to images in their dreams. Dreams seem to be particularly powerful because they deal in images and metaphors, which seem to involve an experiential–intuitive mode of information processing (Epstein, 1994). Hence, working with dreams might actually speed therapy up or help to develop a focus in the therapy. For example, one client presented a dream during a first session that she took her hair off and cooked it in a skillet. By working with this dream, it became evident that she had issues with identity and self-esteem, which might not have surfaced so clearly or quickly without the benefit of the dream interpretation.

Working with a dream using the model proposed in this book usually requires at least a full therapy session and sometimes more. Therapists who are concerned about having just a few sessions in time-limited therapy might at first feel that this amount of time is unwarranted. However, I would note that the time is usually well spent because much personal information that is directly pertinent to the person's major life issues is typically revealed. Because dreams seem to reflect waking issues so poignantly, clients typically talk about issues through this medium that they might not otherwise. Flowers (1993) also noted that clients often express themselves more quickly using the stimulus of dreams than they would otherwise. Similarly, Weiss (1986) and Rosenthal (1980) indicated that dream analysis can help clients reach core issues in psychotherapy quickly, thereby shortening the therapeutic process.

I hope in this book to show that therapists from all orientations can work productively with dreams in either brief or long-term therapy. Furthermore, I hope to show that dreams are important and reflect current conflicts. We seem to dream more when we are under stress, so working with dreams can be a useful method for discovering and reexperiencing feelings, especially when the person is blocked from experiencing his or her feelings.

I do not contend that all dreams need to be discussed in therapy, although it could be useful in very open-ended therapy to discuss as many dreams as possible. Given the reality of brief therapy, however, therapists need to be more selective in deciding which dreams to discuss. It seems particularly important for therapists to be prepared to deal with dreams that are vivid, salient, recurrent, troubling, or reflective of trauma. Clients typically remember these dreams even when they would rather forget them. Thus, rather than worrying about how to get clients to recall their dreams, therapists probably need to pay most attention to those dreams that are brought up spontaneously in therapy. Of course, therapists do need to let clients know that they are willing to work with dreams, or clients may not assume that therapists value dreams.

THERAPIST-GUIDED VERSUS SELF-GUIDED DREAM INTERPRETATION

The focus of this book is on working with dreams in therapy rather than on self-help or learning to interpret dreams by oneself. Working with dreams with a therapist seems to be beneficial because it is often difficult to work with one's own dreams. When working on their own, people often find themselves avoiding difficult areas, discounting painful aspects of dreams, denying that dreams have any meaning, or simply not having the energy or discipline to go through dreams systematically. It is easy to skip important parts of the interpretation process because of the time and energy involved in doing a thorough interpretation. Dreams also often stir up distressing memories that can be painful for people to deal with by themselves. Thus, it is often easier to try to understand dreams with a therapist who can provide the support and encouragement necessary to delve into painful issues. I would recommend that therapists educate their clients about dreams, perhaps by asking them to read this book, so that clients can participate more fully in the interpretation process and can use the skills later to work with dreams on their own.

At the same time, I think that people can probably use this model to explore their own dreams. We are now conducting a study comparing dream interpretation with a therapist to self-help using this model. I would emphasize, however, that working with dreams with an objective, trained therapist can be very beneficial, particularly when one is first learning how to work with dreams; when dreams are recurrent, troubling, or salient; or when the person has a difficult time coming to some understanding on his or her own. The support of another person is invaluable when one is trying to understand oneself. Hence, I highly recommend seeking help from a trained therapist who values dreamwork.

PURPOSE OF THIS BOOK

My general purpose in this book is to present the dream formation and dream interpretation models that I have developed, in collaboration with my students, over a number of years. These models are anchored in the current research and theory on sleep, dreaming, and cognition.

Dream Formation Model

The dream formation model assumes that dreams reflect waking life and are an attempt to integrate waking experiences into existing memory structures (schemata). In brief, events during waking life stimulate relevant schemata. These schemata are thus activated during sleep and, together with the waking events, form the basis of the story (dream) that the dreamer weaves in an attempt to understand current situations in light of past memories. When dreams work, current events are assimilated into memories. However, when waking experiences are too stressful or too discrepant from existing schemata, dreams cannot do their work. Hence, the person has troubled and perhaps recurrent dreams or nightmares.

Dream Interpretation Model

In interpreting dreams, then, we need to reactivate the relevant schemata and attempt to change them so that they can accommodate stressful waking experiences. The dream interpretation model that I propose is an effort to reactivate the schemata through affectively laden associations, change the schemata through insight, and consolidate changes to the schemata through action.

This dream interpretation model is an integration of Freudian, Jungian, experiential, and behavioral theories into a basic three-stage model of therapy proposed by Carkhuff (1969) and Egan (1986). This model assumes that cognitions, experience, insight, and action are all essential components of therapy.

I use a minimal amount of jargon so that the model can be used by therapists from a wide range of theoretical orientations. The model uses common therapist interventions that work well in either short- or long-term approaches. It is a collaborative model that is based on the premise that only the client has the key to the dream and the therapist's job is to work with him or her to decipher the meaning. I believe that dreams are personal and cannot be interpreted with a dream dictionary or standard symbolic interpretations.

The dream interpretation model involves three stages: exploration, insight, and action. In the Exploration Stage, therapists first ask clients to retell the dream. They then go back through the dream sequentially, with clients first describing each image more thoroughly to reimmerse themselves in the experience of the dream, and then associating (saying whatever comes to mind) to the image. Reimmersing themselves in the dream and associating to the images leads directly to the waking conflicts and the associated memories that caused the dreams to occur. Following the thorough exploration of the images, waking conflicts, and memories, the therapist moves to the Insight Stage, in which the therapist facilitates the client in coming to a new understanding of the meaning of the dream. The dream can be understood of several different levels: the dream itself, current waking life, past experiences, or the dream representing parts of oneself. Once the person comes to a new understanding of the dream, the therapist helps the client move to the Action Stage, in which they decide what the client could do differently now that he or she has attained some new self-understanding. Action often arises naturally after exploration and insight but sometimes has to be stimulated by the therapist so that the client does not get stuck in endless experiencing or sterile insight. The action may be related to changing the dream, continued work on the dream, or actual changes in the person's life.

THERAPIST TRAINING

I mentioned earlier that many therapists are reluctant to work with dreams because they have not been trained and are not sure what to do with dreams. Therapists can easily learn to use the model presented in this book to work with clients' dreams. To learn the model, I first recommend that therapists read this book (and other dream interpretation books) carefully. Second, therapists should ideally attend a workshop with someone who teaches and demonstrates dream interpretation. Third, therapists can work through several of their own dreams using the self-guided manual presented at the end of the book. Going through one's own dreams using this approach really begins to provide an idea of how to do it. Fourth, therapists can participate in peer supervision groups, which provide wonderful opportunities to review one's work with dream interpretation as well as to analyze each other's dreams using the model. Interpreting one's own dreams is probably the most effective way to learn to use the model and to experience it personally—personal experience is powerful proof of the efficacy of dream interpretation. We have found peer supervision groups to be effective in teaching the principles of dream interpretation and also to be a very exciting and stimulating experience for all involved. Finally, I recommend doing many supervised sessions. The major factor that seems to help therapists learn this model is a good deal of practice with a lot of feedback about performance in each stage.

FORMAT OF THE BOOK

In the first part of the book, I present background material that is useful for understanding the origins of this dream interpretation model. Chapter 2 presents a brief review of the theory and research on sleep and dreaming, focusing on what therapists need to know to be able to place clients' experiences into a normative framework. For example, they need to know about the causes of recurrent dreams and sleep terrors. They also need to know when to refer clients for the assessment and treatment of sleep disorders. Chapter 3 presents a brief overview of dream interpretation from ancient times to the present. Again, an understanding of the different views about dreams and the different methods that have been used to deal with dreams is informative for therapists. People who are familiar with the research and history and/or who are eager first to learn more about the present model might want to skip over these foundation chapters and go straight to the chapters presenting the dream formation and dream interpretation models.

Chapter 4 presents the cognitive–experiential model of dreams and dream interpretation. Understanding the origins and functions of dreams sets the stage for how to work with dreams. For example, the theory that dreams reflect an attempt to integrate waking issues into memories of previous experiences dictates a personal rather than a symbolic approach to dream interpretation. Chapter 5 presents the theory and guidelines for implementing the Exploration Stage (including the steps of retelling the dream, reimmersing the client in the experience of the dream, exploring the images of the dream from an affective and cognitive perspective, linking the images to waking life, and working with the affect and conflicts raised by the exploration). Chapter 6 presents the theory and guidelines for implementing the Insight Stage (which involves trying to understand the meaning of the dream). Chapter 7 presents the theory and guidelines for implementing the Action Stage (which involves deciding what to do differently on the basis of the dream interpretation). Therapeutic issues that arise in using the model (choosing which dreams to interpret and with whom to use dream interpretation, introducing dreams in therapy, using dreams at specific times in therapy, using dream images as metaphors in therapy after the dream interpretation, monitoring client responsiveness to dream interpretation, maintaining flexibility, and dealing with countertransference issues) are presented in Chapter 8.

The third section of the book provides extended examples from clinical practice of how to do dream interpretation using this model. An example of a single-session dream interpretation is presented in Chapter 9. In Chapter 10, recurrent dreams and nightmares are discussed, along with an extended example of working with a recurrent dream in individual therapy. Chapter 11 describes the model as applied to dream groups, along with an extended example of a session of a dream group for recently separated and divorcing women.

The fourth section deals with research on dreams and therapy. A review of the empirical literature, along with ideas for future research on dream interpretation, is presented in Chapter 12. I would like to encourage more researchers to study dream interpretation, perhaps using this book as a manualized approach, so that we can learn more about the effects of dream interpretation.

Finally, a self-guided manual for dream interpretation is presented in the Appendix. Therapists can use this manual as an adjunct in therapy; for example, after going through a dream interpretation session with a client, therapists might ask clients to work with another dream on their own for more practice and then bring the results back for discussion in therapy.

❦ CHAPTER TWO

Sleep and Dreaming

T O WORK WITH dreams in therapy, therapists need to have at least a minimal understanding of sleep and dreams at both a physiological and psychological level. This chapter offers an overview of the research on the physiology of sleep and dreaming, recall of dreams, dream content, and functions of dreams.

PHYSIOLOGY OF SLEEP AND DREAMING[1]

As the average adult gets ready for sleep, he or she goes into a hypnogogic reverie where thoughts are loosely connected but relatively similar to waking thoughts. From this reverie, the person descends into sleep, progressing from light sleep (stage 1) to deep sleep (stage 4). Each of the first four stages of sleep has characteristic brain wave patterns that become slower with each stage. In addition, respiration and heart rate slow down progressively in each stage, such that rousing a person from stage 4 sleep is particularly difficult. People do often engage in mentation during these four stages of non-rapid-eye-movement (NREM) sleep, and much of this mental activity qualifies as dreaming. Mentation during NREM sleep, however, is not recalled as readily, is

---

[1]This section summarizes the research and writing on sleep and sleep deprivation. by several authors (Antrobus, Antrobus, & Fisher, 1965; Aserinsky & Kleitman, 1953, 1955; Cartwright & Lamberg, 1992; Dement, 1955; Dement & Kleitman, 1957a, 1957b; Dement & Wolpert, 1958; Foulkes, 1964, 1985a, 1985b; Foulkes & Vogel, 1965; R. Greenberg & Pearlman, 1993; Gross et al., 1966; Herman, Roffwarg, & Tauber, 1968; Hobson, 1988; Hobson & McCarley, 1977; Kales, Malstrom, Kee, Kales, & Tan, 1969; Kleitman, 1963; Koulack, 1991; Monroe, Rechtschaffen, Foulkes, & Jensen, 1965; Rechtschaffen & Buchignani, 1983; Rechtschaffen, Verdone, & Wheaton, 1963; Snyder, 1970; Starker, 1973; W. B. Webb & Kersey, 1967).

less vivid and visual, seems to be more like thinking and less like dreaming, and is concerned more directly with waking life than thinking (dreams) that occurs during rapid-eye-movement (REM) sleep (the fifth stage).

After about 30–40 minutes of stage 4 sleep, a person typically turns over or shifts about and then begins ascending back through stages 3 and 2. The person then goes into the fifth stage, or what has been called REM sleep or paradoxical sleep because it is very different from the other stages of sleep. Respiration and heart rate become more irregular, the larger muscles of the body become immobile except for twitches in the extremities, men and women become sexually aroused, brain waves become faster, the person can be roused relatively easily, and the person begins having bursts of eye movements (called rapid eye movements or REM). The REM state originates in the brainstem. Cholinergic neurons fire during REM, and other neurons associated with attentional processes (using the transmitters norepinephrine and serotonin) turn off during sleep, causing remote memories to be more easily accessed. Dreams tend to be relatively vivid, hallucinatory, visual experiences that are charged with emotion. About 60–90% of people who are awakened from REM sleep can recall their dreams.

Most dreams from REM sleep reflect the colors of the everyday world, although dreams seem to be a bit darker and more out of focus than perception in waking life. Typically, the better the dream recall, the more likely it is that dreamers will report color in the dream. REM dreams seem to be in color more often than NREM dreams.

People cycle through each of the five stages of sleep approximately every 90 minutes. In the early part of the night, more time is spent in the deeper stages of sleep with only about 10 minutes spent in REM sleep. During each successive 90-minute period, less time is spent in stages 3 and 4 and more time is spent in REM sleep, so that the person might be spending up to an hour of the last cycle in REM sleep. A person who sleeps between 6 and 9 hours a night typically has between four to six REM periods, involving anywhere from an 1½ to 2 hours or about 20–25% of the total sleep time.

Dreams appear to be part of a 24-hour cognitive arousal cycle that continues in wakefulness. Some sort of dreaming activity seems to be present throughout waking and sleeping states, with daydream content similar to nightdream content. Hence, daydreams could be just as important to examine in therapy as night dreams.

We tend not to remember our dreams in the morning, perhaps because the norepinephrine and serotonin that would imprint them in long-term memory are not active during the REM state. This inability to recall dreams has obvious implications for using dreams in therapy. If people cannot recall dreams, it is not possible to work with them in dream interpretation.

REM sleep seems to be necessary for higher order cognitive tasks.

Memory for simple word lists does not seem to be affected by REM deprivation, but performance on creative thinking and problem-solving tasks is impaired by REM deprivation. Furthermore, it appears that REM sleep increases when learning is taking place, suggesting that REM sleep helps people incorporate new learning. So, in fact, it seems that it does help to "sleep on it."

Children and the elderly appear to have different patterns of sleep and dreaming. Children have substantially more REM sleep, whereas the elderly have substantially less REM sleep.

In addition, some people suffer from sleepwalking (which typically occurs during deep NREM sleep), in which they have minimal ability to control their behaviors. Others suffer from night terrors (also called sleep terrors), which are sudden arousals usually during NREM sleep with blood-curdling screams or crying, often accompanied by signs of intense fear. Both sleepwalking and sleep terrors are common in preadolescent children, particularly in those who are late bedwetters. Sleepwalking and sleep terrors seem to be associated with trouble shifting from NREM sleep to REM sleep. Heavy exercise, a loss of sleep over a few nights, or extreme stress can exacerbate problems with sleepwalking and sleep terrors. Some people have REM sleep behavior disorder, a problem in which the large muscles are not paralyzed so that the person actually acts out his or her dreams, sometimes resulting in disastrous consequences (such as murder). Some people lose the paralysis of the muscles during REM sleep as they age, which in the past has been misdiagnosed as serious mental illness because of the resulting thrashing about during sleep. Still others have paralysis of the large muscles outside of REM sleep, causing them to feel like their bodies are not under their own control.

Alcohol typically reduces the amount of time spent in REM sleep and the amount of eye movements associated with REM sleep. When the alcohol is withdrawn, REM usually rebounds such that REM sleep occurs in abnormally high amounts. The accompanying dreams tend to be intense and unpleasant. Some types of sleeping pills have the same effects as alcohol on REM sleep, although other types are specifically designed not to interfere with REM sleep.

Stress also seems to have a profound effect on dreams. When people have been shown stressful movies prior to sleep, their dreams clearly indicated incorporation of the stressful stimuli (Baekeland, Koulack, & Lasky, 1968; Cartwright, Kasniak, Borowitz, & Kling, 1972; Goodenough, Witkin, Koulack, & Cohen, 1975). In addition, people involved in stressful group therapy sessions showed changes in dream content (Breger, Hunter, & Lane, 1971). These results indicate that presleep experiences altered the content of dreams and the accompanying mood. Thus, stress events have a greater impact on dreams than neutral or benign events (Koulack, 1991). From their research, Piccione, Jacobs, Kramer, and Roth (1977) concluded that dreams were most likely to incorporate the daytime activity with the most intense emotional tone.

Implications for Therapists

1. Therapists need to be aware, at least minimally, of the normal patterns of sleep so that they can assess whether their clients' sleep patterns are disturbed.
2. Therapists need to be aware that sleep disturbances and sleep deprivation can create serious problems.
3. Therapists would be well advised to include questions about sleep in routine history and assessment batteries so that they can make accurate assessments about the origins of problems.
4. If a therapist suspects that a client has a sleep disorder, the therapist should refer the client for an assessment in a sleep laboratory; sleep laboratories are often available at local hospitals.
5. Therapists need to be aware of the effects of alcohol, sleeping pills, and medications on REM sleep and recommend adjustments in dosages if necessary.

FUNCTIONS OF DREAMS

At this point, no one knows for certain why we dream, but many theories about the function of dreams have been advanced. Some theories suggest that the function of dreams is the expression of unconscious wishes, others suggest that the function is physiological, and still others that the function is process information and/or emotions.

Expression of Unconscious Wishes

Hippocrates and Plato both believed in the psychological function of dreams. Plato thought that when our reasoning ability was suspended during sleep, passions and desires revealed themselves with full force. Likewise, Freud (1900/1966) hypothesized that dreams resulted from psychological events. He thought that dreams were instigated by unconscious, unacceptable wishes that arise during sleep. He suggested that wishes are made more acceptable by distortions that disguise their true nature. Thus, according to Freud, dreams serve as disguised wish fulfillments. Freud also suggested that dreams function to preserve sleep by decreasing the growing tension created by the unfulfilled wishes. If dreams express unconscious wishes, dreams may indeed serve as the royal road to uncovering hidden desires and fears in therapy. Unfortunately, minimal evidence has been found to support Freud's hypotheses.

Physiological Functions

In opposition to Freud's theory, Hobson and McCarley proposed a controversial activation–synthesis hypothesis about dreaming based on recent research in the neurobiology of dreaming (Hobson, 1988; Hobson, Hoffman, Heflan, & Kostner, 1987; Hobson & McCarley, 1977; McCarley & Hobson, 1977; McCarley & Hoffman, 1981). They proposed that physiological events during REM sleep explain the occurrence and unique characteristics of dreams. REM sleep is generated by electrical activity of neurons in the pons, which is located in the hindbrain. The pontine neurons that generate REM sleep randomly send electrical signals to many brain areas including the forebrain, which is responsible for thoughts, sensations, and feelings. According to the activation–synthesis hypothesis, the activation of the forebrain areas generates the conscious dream experience. Thus, the random activation produces a number of images, thoughts, feelings, and memories that the forebrain synthesizes into a narrative. The forebrain does the best it can to integrate all the pieces together into a cohesive whole, but dream distortion comes about because of the brain's incapacity to synthesize all the random patterns of activation. Thus, Hobson and McCarley suggest that dreams are stimulated by physiological events rather than being the result of meaningful psychological events such as the fulfillment of unconscious wishes.

The frequency of visual and auditory sensations and limb movements in dreams, as well as the occurrence of distortion and bizarre images provide support for the activation–synthesis hypothesis (Vogel, 1978, 1993). Further, the activation–synthesis hypothesis suggests that REM dream properties are consistent with physiological events during REM sleep (Vogel, 1978, 1993). However, whereas the activation-synthesis hypothesis would predict that dreams should be almost a kaleidoscopic sequence of meaningless images, dreams usually are coherent narratives, are not bizarre, and are related to waking life. Thus, rather than people imposing meaning on seemingly unrelated images in dreams, dreams seem to be meaningful from the beginning.

Another theory is that dreams serve a restorative function. According to this theory, dreaming may give the noncentral nervous system a break for restorative purposes and to keep the mind warm so that it can work efficiently when awake (Antrobus, 1993). In other words, dreaming might keep the mind active during sleep, with the alternation between REM and NREM sleep being necessary to give both systems rest and activation (Globus, 1993). REM might help to modulate intentions, instincts, and affects so that the cognitive networks are open to wider possibilities on waking (Globus, 1993).

Crick and Mitchison (1983) proposed that dreaming serves the function of ridding the brain of irrelevant material. They suggested that people dream to forget and that dreaming is essentially the wastebasket of the brain. During REM sleep, they postulated that the brain eliminates mental activity that might interfere with rational thought and activity. The waking brain makes more connections between brain cells than are needed for efficient memory and thinking, so the dream's function is to clear the brain of these unneeded, meaningless connections. In their conceptualization, REM is essentially a random unlearning that prunes overcrowded networks. Their theory suggests that it might actually be damaging to recall one's dreams because doing so might strengthen neural connections that should be purged.

Information-Processing Theories

Another theory is that dreaming is a meaningful, motivated activity, involved in matching current experiences with past experiences in long-term memory and integrating this new information into organized memory structures (Palombo, 1978, 1980, 1987). The research about the importance of dreaming for helping people remember provides support for this theory (see the review by R. Greenberg & Pearlman, 1993). Similarly, Evans (1983) proposed that dreams allow an opportunity to integrate the day's experiences with memories stored in the brain. They further contended that one need not disturb this process by recalling dreams.

Emotion-Processing Theories

Breger (1967, 1969) postulated that dreaming serves the distinctive role of processing emotional information. He proposed that dreaming is necessary to assimilate (incorporate and organize) new experience into affective memory schemata that have successfully handled such data in the past. Breger viewed dreaming as an assimilative form of thought, allowing free experimentation with problem situations. From these situations, fantasies emerge that produce creative solutions. He suggested that the dream state offers advantages over the waking state for dealing with emotional material. In effect, he stated that memory systems are creatively opened up given that stored information is more accessible during dreaming because of minimal demands from the external environment. He noted that associational processes are more fluid, social acceptability pressures are minimized, and more ways of manipulating linguistic and perceptual symbols are available during dreaming.

Breger (1969) hypothesized that emotionally laden events in waking life activate memories of previously evocative events and thus stimulate dreams during sleep. Thus, dream meaning depends on the structure of one's memory networks, especially those related to affect. Breger does not suggest that dreams will necessarily yield good solutions to problems, but that the process of integrating the conflictual material during dreaming provides a cathartic function that allows one to awaken psychologically refreshed the next morning.

Dreams also might serve an accommodative function (such that the dreamer is changed as a result of the dream experience) in addition to an assimilative function (in which new information is incorporated) (Cartwright, 1986; Kramer, 1992). Kramer (1992) posited that 60% of dreams function automatically, outside of conscious awareness, in an assimilative manner. With these "successful" dreams, sleep proceeds relatively free of disturbance and there is no memory of dreams in the waking state. The accommodative dream, however, is more likely to be recalled and must then be understood to exert its transformative effects. This type of dream has the potential to exert a significant impact on the dreamer's life. Kramer's (1982) selective mood regulatory theory of dreaming is based on the findings that intense emotional waking experiences, especially from interpersonal situations, structure the content of dreams. Kramer proposed that dreams act to contain the affective surge that occurs during REM sleep.

The occurrence of posttraumatic stress disorder (PTSD) and recurrent dreams provides support for the theory that dreams serve an emotion-processing function (Domhoff, 1993). PTSD dreams replay the actual traumatic event, often causing the person to wake up in terror. In contrast, recurrent dreams seem to be watered-down versions of PTSD dreams and nightmares, such that the exact event is not replayed but the theme is replayed in a more metaphorical form. Domhoff suggests that nightmares and recurrent dreams represent the failure of the dream to be able to deal with the traumatic events. In usual circumstances, a person is able to use his or her dreams to process the emotional information that comes up during the day, but dreams seem to be unable to process extraordinarily traumatic events. Cartwright and Lamberg (1992) suggested that the dream function gets stuck and is unable to do the job of helping the person integrate the traumatic event.

Multipurpose Functions of Dreams

Boss (1958, 1977) argued that all experiential modalities of human existence potentially exist in dreaming. He suggested that there is not a single fundamental function of dreaming, any more than there is a fundamental function for human existence in general. Hunt (1989) agreed that there is no single deep structure to dreams. In fact, he argued that dreams serve many different purposes precisely because they have no fixed function. He proposed several overlapping categories of dreams: mundane dreams, Freudian-type pressure-discharge dreams, dreams based on somatic states and illnesses, dreams based on metaphor, dreams based on problem solving and deep intuition, lucid-control dreams, various types of nightmares, and Jungian archetypal-mythological dreams. He proposed that the mundane dreams serve to consolidate and reorganize memories.

Summary

A number of theories have been proposed to explain the functions of dreams. These theories variously suggest that the function of dreams is wish fulfillment, the preservation of sleep, physiological excitation, information processing of waking events, or emotional processing of waking events. At this point, we do not have conclusive evidence regarding the function of dreams, but it seems most likely that dreams serve a variety of functions (Hunt, 1989). I personally have a hard time believing that something as rich and creative as dreams serves no particular function. It seems more likely that there is some physiological or sensory function (e.g., random bursts or keeping parts of the brain "warm"), but that there are also psychological functions such as problem solving. Certainly dreams can have both physiological and psychological functions concurrently. The theory that makes most sense to me is that dreams are an attempt to process information and resolve emotional preoccupations. The similarity of dreams to waking events (discussed later in this chapter) provides evidence for this theory.

Antrobus (1993), Domhoff (1993), and Hunt (1986) have all argued that even if dreams have no psychological function, the analysis of dreams that are recalled can still be quite beneficial. Because dreams (perhaps serendipitously) reflect waking life, they can be used for greater self-understanding. Hence, regardless of the ultimate discovery about "the" function(s) of dreams, I believe that therapists are justified in working with dreams in therapy because (1) they reflect concerns from waking life, and (2) they seem to serve a function of helping us cope with and integrate information and emotions.

RECALL OF DREAMS

Although almost everyone dreams several dreams per night, only a few dreams are recalled upon waking. Variables related to the dream itself, the personality of the dreamer, and the situation all influence dream recall.

Salient dreams, or those that are novel, bizarre, vivid, active, long, and emotionally charged, are more likely to be remembered than bland dreams (Cartwright, 1977, 1979; Cohen, 1974a, 1974b; Kramer, 1982; Meier, Ruell, Ziegler, & Hall, 1968; Trinder & Kramer, 1971). Dreams tend to be more salient and emotionally charged when stressful events have taken place during the preceding day (Koulack, 1991). When we feel emotionally charged during the day, we are likely to dream about these events in a way such that our dreams are more emotionally charged, and then we are more likely to recall these dreams in the morning. Thus, there seems to be some continuity between our waking experiences and the content of our dreams.

Position of dreams during the night also influences recall. The final dreams of the night are the most easily remembered (Trinder & Kramer, 1971), perhaps because of their recency upon awakening. Interference also diminishes one's recall of dreams because dreamers become distracted from their dreams upon awakening (Cohen & Wolfe, 1973; Goodenough, 1978). However, rehearsing dreams upon awakening can aid in memory (Koulack & Goodenough, 1976). In addition, arousal while a dream is taking place allows a person to rehearse it and thus to store it in long-term memory. So if you wake up in the middle of the night to go to the bathroom and rehearse the dream, you will be more likely to remember it in the morning. Because dreams that have high degrees of emotion are often associated with brief periods of arousal, these dreams are most likely to be remembered (Koulack, 1991). Light sleepers also seem to recall their dreams more easily, perhaps because they are nearer to the waking state.

Dreams are recalled more often by women than men (Carrington, 1972; Winget, Kramer, & Whitman, 1972) and more by introverts than extroverts (Cann & Donderi, 1986; Cartwright, 1977; A. B. Hill, 1974; Lewis, Goodenough, Shapiro, & Sleser, 1966; Wallach, 1963). Dream recall also appears to be related to cognitive style, particularly such variables as divergent thinking, associative productivity, imagistic ability, and richness of inner life (Cohen, 1974b). In addition, a positive attitude toward dreams and a belief in their meaningfulness have been shown to correlate with high recall ability (Cartwright, 1978; Cohen, 1974b; Garfield, 1974). Finally, where the dream is experienced and collected, how the dreamer awakens, how dream reports are collected, the time of night and stage of sleep at which the dreamer awakens, how the dream is recorded, and the sleeping habits of the dreamer all influence dream recall (Cartwright, 1977; Kramer, 1982).

Suggestions for Improving Dream Recall

Several books have offered ideas for helping people remember their dreams (Cartwright & Lamberg, 1992; Delaney, 1988; Faraday, 1974; Garfield, 1974), including the following:

1. Avoid alcohol because it reduces REM sleep.
2. Instruct yourself to remember your dreams before going to sleep. Believing that dreams are valuable seems to increase the probability of recall.
3. Keep a notebook (and perhaps a lighted pen) next to your bed and write down dreams as soon as you awaken, even if it is in the middle of the night. Some people prefer to speak their dreams into a recorder that they keep right next to their bed because it doesn't wake them up as much. Then they transcribe the dream in the morning.
4. Sleep as long as you can because you spend more time in REM sleep the longer you sleep.
5. Waking without an alarm allows some people to move gradually from the dream state into the waking state. This gradual wakening sometimes strengthens the probability of remembering the dream.
6. Staying in the body position you were in during the dream can sometimes facilitate recall.
7. Rehearse the dream before getting up. Perhaps try to fix on a key image to help you remember.
8. Don't pressure yourself to remember your dreams. Sometimes when you try too hard, dreams vanish. Not everyone recalls their dreams, so dream interpretation will not be an appropriate intervention for everyone.

Issues about the Accuracy of Dream Reports

The dream as it is related later may be quite different than the dream that actually occurred. Two things might happen to change the dream content. First, people typically forget all but the most salient and vivid dreams upon awakening (Koulack, 1991). Details are lost unless the dream is rehearsed or written down immediately. Second, as time progresses and the person thinks about the dream, he or she may elaborate upon it to make it more logical or palatable, often not even being aware that the meaning is changing. Loftus (1988) noted that memory for waking events is very imperfect and susceptible to external influences. Probably memory for dreams is even more susceptible to external influence because dreams are so fleeting and not always logical. I should note that there are many theories and a great deal of controversy over how memories in general are stored and retrieved.

Some evidence for the selectivity of dream report was found by Whitman, Kramer, and Baldridge (1963). They obtained dream reports from two people in a sleep laboratory and then studied which dreams the people chose to report later to a psychiatrist. Dreams that the people thought might elicit a negative response from the psychiatrist (e.g., of sexuality) were not reported. Thus, clients may well alter their dreams to meet with therapist approval. Reassuring clients that whatever they report is acceptable is undoubtedly important so as to permit clients to tell their dreams (and waking issues) to therapists.

DREAM CONTENT

Dream content refers to what is overtly present in the dream report. Dream content can be observed by anyone. In contrast, dream interpretation refers to the attempt to try to understand the meaning of the dream for the individual (see also Jones, 1970, for distinctions between dream investigation and dream interpretation).

Some types of dreams are very common or typical. People from all over the world have reported having chase dreams, falling dreams, flying dreams, and nudity dreams (Griffith, Miyago, & Tago, 1958; Harris, 1948; Hall, 1955; Kramer, Winget, & Whitman, 1971). Delaney (1991) reported several common dream themes, although some of these may be specific to the American culture: teeth falling out; chase and pursuit dreams; falling; nudity; being barefoot; flying; missing the boat, train, or bus; losing one's purse, wallet, keys, or briefcase; finding money or lost treasure; dreams of being in bed with an unexpected partner; having parents observe your lovemaking; trying to find a private toilet; examination dreams; being unable to run or call out for help; dreams of discovering that you have been neglecting or starving little animals; mourning dreams; and talking animals.

Hall (1947, 1953) believed that dreams are projections of personality dynamics and that a close examination of written dream reports permits a scientific investigation of personality. He analyzed the content of 10,000 written dream reports of college students (Hall, 1953). The characters in the dreams were usually people with whom the dreamer was emotionally and often conflictually involved. The settings were generally commonplace and familiar (e.g., a house, car, street) and involved recreation more often than work. Most of the activity involved some sort of movement like walking or climbing but also involved passive activities like talking. In keeping with the cultural norms of the era, he found that women engaged in more passive activities than did men in their dreams. Although emotionally varied, dream content showed twice as many negative emotions (e.g., fear, anger, and sadness) as positive emotions (e.g., happiness). Hall's research led him to conclude that dreams revealed attempts to resolve current conflicts rather than representing repressed infantile or Oedipal drives, as Freud believed.

In a more extensive analysis of 1,000 dreams, Hall and Van de Castle (1966) found that women recalled dreams an average of 8% more often than men and that women's dreams had more emotional content. Women usually had more indoor settings with household articles in their dreams, and more body parts and clothing. Women also had more characters in their dreams, and these characters were equally often men and women. Women's dreams were more often of familiar people and more often of children and babies. The encounters that women had in their dreams were more often friendly and their sexual encounters were with familiar men.

In contrast, men's dreams involved more outdoor settings with tools, weapons, and recreational items. Men's dreams involved more explicit sex, money, men, unfamiliar people, animals, and sexual encounters with unfamiliar women. An equal amount of aggression was shown, although women's dreams involved more nonphysical aggression than did men's. As in Hall (1953), negative emotions predominated over positive emotions for both men and women.

Subsequent studies (Cartwright, Lloyd, Knight, & Trenholme, 1984; Cohen, 1973; Lortie-Lussier, Schwab, & deKonick, 1985) have found that dream content for women has changed since Hall and Van de Castle's early work. For example, Lortie-Lussier et al. (1985) found that the dreams of working women involved more unpleasant emotions, more male characters, less overt hostility, and fewer residential dream settings than did those of homemakers. As societal roles and expectations for women have changed, women's dreams also seem to have changed, reflecting their activities in waking life. The changes in dream content for women over time are particularly interesting and again suggest that dreams closely mirror waking lives.

Marital status, racial/ethnic background, socioeconomic status, and developmental stage also seem to influence dream content. For example, women in the midst of divorce have been shown to have dreams reflecting their waking reactions to the divorce (Cartwright et al., 1984). Winget et al. (1972) found that divorced and widowed persons had more death concerns in their dreams than did single or married persons, Euro-Americans had more covert hostility than African-Americans, people from lower socioeconomic classes had more characters in their dreams than did people from upper classes, and young adults had more guilt whereas elderly people had more death anxiety in their dreams. LeVine (1966) found differing amounts of achievement imagery in boys from three different Nigerian tribes that mirrored the differential power systems of the tribes. Roll, Hinton, and Glazer (1974) found more images of death in dreams of Mexican-American students, especially the women, than Anglo-American students. Children's dreams typically involved figures, settings, and actions familiar in their waking lives, with a preponderance of animal characters and friendly social interactions (Foulkes, 1985a; Foulkes, Hollifield, Sullivan, Bradley, & Terry, 1990).

Dreams also appear to be related to pathology. Dreams of depressed people were found to be full of masochism, dependency needs, and self-defeating thoughts and ideas (Beck & Hurvich, 1959; Beck & Ward, 1961; Cartwright, 1986; Kramer, Whitman, Baldridge, & Lansky, 1966). Schizophrenics' dreams were filled with feelings of loneliness, a lack of human contact, sterility, limited and/or bizarre imagery, danger, morbidity, a sense of emergency or stress, and feelings of hopelessness and helplessness (Biddle, 1963; Carrington, 1972; Dement, 1955; Kant, 1942; Noble, 1951). Dreams of hysterics were characterized by poor impulse control, exhibitionism, and aggressive sexual acting out; paranoid schizophrenics' dreams had paranoid and delusionary thinking; and psychotically depressed persons' dreams were filled with hopelessness, sadness, and loss of self-esteem (Langs, 1966). Dreams of chronic brain syndrome patients were less complex, involved fewer people and objects, and contained fewer and simpler actions and interactions than did those of normal people (Kramer & Roth, 1979). Finally, dreams of sex offenders contained stronger sexual elements than did those of other criminals (Goldhirsch, 1961).

Dream content also has been shown to vary with medication (Cartwright, 1966; Kramer, Whitman, Baldridge, & Ornstein, 1970) and with waking mood change (Cartwright et al., 1984). In addition, dream content can be manipulated by presleep suggestion (Cartwright, 1974) and hypnosis (Reichers, Kramer, & Trinder, 1970). Researchers have often been incorporated into dream content when people sleep in sleep laboratories (Barad, Altschuler, & Goldfarb, 1961), with the gender of the researcher influencing the content of dreams (Fox, Kramer, Baldridge, Whitman, & Ornstein, 1968).

Finally, dreams seem to reflect current waking concerns. Cartwright (1979) suggested that dreams tend to be more vivid and more easily recalled during times of increased emotional stress and upset moods such as during a divorce transition. Cartwright et al. (1984), for example, showed that divorcing women dreamed about divorce whereas nondivorcing women did not. Trenholme, Cartwright, and Greenberg (1984) found that divorcing women's dreams contained more themes of being threatened and ridiculed, with a more urgent need for harm avoidance, than did the dreams of a stably married cohort. Similarly, Garfield (1991) found that dreams of being buried alive or lost at sea were common for women anticipating or undergoing divorce. The dreams presented at the beginning of Chapter 1 provide examples of the incorporation of divorce themes into dreams in our study of dream groups for recently separated and divorcing women (Falk & Hill, 1995).

A central conclusion from these studies on dream content is that dreamers usually dream about what is going on in their waking lives. These findings give credence to the "continuity hypothesis" (Adler, 1936; Cartwright, 1969; Cohen, 1973; Hall, 1953; Hall & Nordby, 1972;

Kramer, Hlasny, Jacobs, & Roth, 1976) that dreams are meaningful, organized, and nonrandom events that reflect the personality and waking life rather than disguise waking concerns.

Implications for Therapists

The content of dreams can give therapists clues about what is going on in clients' lives. For example, if a client's dreams are filled with masochism, dependency, and self-defeating thoughts and ideas, therapists should be alerted to look for other signs of depression. However, I would caution therapists against interpreting dreams strictly on the basis of overt content without the dreamer's associations. For example, although women going through separation or divorce may be more likely than nondivorcing women to dream about being buried alive or being lost at sea, these images might have different meanings for each person. Using an actuarial approach to dream interpretation loses the richness and individuality of the dream process. I would emphasize that only the dreamer has the key to the dream interpretation.

SUMMARY

Empirical investigations in sleep and dreaming indicate that there are 90-minute cycles during sleep with people cycling through five stages and spending progressively more time during each cycle in REM sleep. The average person spends about 2 to 2½ hours per night in REM sleep (when most of the dreaming occurs). Although virtually everyone dreams, not all dreams are recalled. Furthermore, dreams appear to be meaningful, consistent with personality structures, and connected to events in waking life. Most researchers and theorists, even those who are psychoanalytic, now believe that dreams do not disguise waking issues but rather reflect them. Thus, dreams seem to be metaphorical attempts to deal with current experiences and emotional preoccupations. We can conclude that, although no one knows for certain why we dream or what the functions of dreams are, examining dreams can be helpful because they reflect waking concerns.

CHAPTER THREE

History of Dream Interpretation

N EW IDEAS and theories rarely, if ever, arise in a vacuum, but rather are a new integration of old theories. Hence, it is useful, before venturing on to a new theory, to explicate the history of ideas in an area. In this chapter, I briefly cover the history of dream interpretation from the time of the first written records. I focus first on methods of dream interpretation from ancient times to the Freudian era,[1] then discuss the early psychoanalytic theories, and finally describe some current theories that have been influential in developing the model presented in this book.

ANCIENT HISTORY

Dreams had a prominent place in the writings of the ancient world. The earliest evidence of interest in dream interpretation comes from clay tablets dating to about 3000 B.C. that contain interpretations about the dreams of Mesopotamians. There were three types of early dreams: message dreams, mantic dreams, and symbolic dreams. Message dreams were experienced by kings, often following incubation rituals in a special temple. A deity or its representative would appear at a king's head and give a personally significant message. Mantic dreams were prophetic dreams, in which one's personal destiny was revealed through signs or "omina." For example, negative dream content was attributed to spirits of the dead and demons, flying dreams indicated disaster,

---

[1]This section summarizes the history of dreams as presented by several authors (Bynum, 1993; Delaney, 1993; Garfield, 1974; Hill, 1996; Kilborne, 1990; Koulack, 1991; Krippner, 1990a, 1990b, 1990c; Savary, 1990; Van de Castle, 1994; W. B. Webb, 1990, 1993). I especially recommend the Van de Castle book to those who want more background because it is a thorough, scholarly treatise on the history of dreams.

drinking wine predicted a short life, and drinking water forecast a long life. Symbolic dreams involved interactions with gods, stars, people, or objects and seemed to express the dreamer's personality dynamics. Symbolic dreams were considered dangerous and indicative of disease or evil; they were not discussed or recorded for fear of increasing their potency. Amulets and charms were used to protect people from bad dreams; rituals were used to ward off the evil consequences of bad dreams. Thus, dreams were a dual-edged sword: they could solve problems but could bring evil consequences.

Similarly, Egyptians interpreted dreams as being messages from the gods. Egyptian dream books from about 2000 B.C. listed types of dreams and suggested what each type meant for the future of the dreamer. Serapis was the Egyptian god of dreams, and serapims were dream temples where people went to have dreams induced.

The earliest Greek view was that a god made a visit during a dream, much like the message dreams of the Mesopotamians. The Greeks also thought that sleeping in special temples and going through elaborate rituals allowed people to gain access to dreams that foretold the future or prescribed cures for illnesses. Many Greeks went to Epidaurus seeking mental, physical, and spiritual healing from Aesclepius, a physician/god. They spent their days in intellectual and emotional activity and in physical healing and nurturing, and spent their nights in dream temples waiting for a healing dream. The dream was expected to offer direction for further treatment or a new glimpse of reality. The next morning the dreams were shared with other dreamers who stayed at the temple.

The views of several early Greeks have been influential even into modern times. Interestingly, a number of different viewpoints were held about dreams. Hippocrates believed that the sense organs were predominant during the day but the emphasis shifted to the soul during dreams. He believed in prophetic, diagnostic, and psychologically revealing dreams. Plato thought that our reasoning ability was suspended during sleep and thus passions and desires revealed themselves with full force. In contrast, Aristotle believed that dreams were merely due to sensory sensations and somatic disturbances. In about 100 A.D., Artemidorus wrote *Oneirocritica* (The Interpretation of Dreams), which can be considered the great-grandfather of all dream books. At the same time that he presented a thorough taxonomy of dreams, Artemidorus urged flexibility in interpreting dreams for the individual dreamer. When the history of dream interpretation is examined, it quickly becomes apparent that Freud and Jung were more the restorers of dream interpretation as it existed in the Greek times rather than the developers of new theories.

Romans were generally influenced by the Greek beliefs and had several shrines for dream incubation. Cicero, however, in a manner similar to Aristotle, believed that dreams were not from the gods. If the gods were truly trying to help people, Cicero argued that they would send the messages when people were awake and better able to receive the information, rather than when people were asleep and prone to forget what they had experienced.

Reference to dreams can also be found in some of the major religious writings of ancient times. The Babylonian Talmud, compiled between 200 B.C. and 200 A.D., had 270 references to dreams. The most quoted saying from the Talmud is from Rabbi Hisda who said, "An uninterpreted dream is like an unread letter." Rabbi Johnathon said, "A man is shown in his dreams what he thinks in his heart." The Old and New Testaments of the Bible have many accounts of the work of dream interpreters in decoding prophetic dreams. For example, in the Old Testament, Joseph interpreted the Pharaoh's dream of the seven fat cattle and seven lean cattle as predicting that there would be seven prosperous years followed by seven years of famine. Because of this dream interpretation, the Pharaoh saved grain during the prosperous years and was able to avoid starvation for his people during the famine that followed. Needless to say, the Pharaoh favored Joseph and rewarded him handsomely for his interpretive ability.

Dream "dictionaries" have also been found in India and China. The sacred Vedas of India, written between 1500 and 1000 B.C., gave specific interpretations of dreams (e.g., to ride an elephant was lucky, whereas riding a donkey was unlucky). Dreams from earlier in the night were thought to not come true for a year, whereas those from the latter part of the night were already half realized. If several dreams were remembered from a night's sleep, only the last was to be interpreted. Evil spirits were to be dispelled with various verses or through rites of purification or baths.

The earliest reference to dreams in China was in 1020 B.C. in the T'ung Shu. The Chinese thought that the soul temporarily left the body to communicate with the dead during dreams. Dreadful consequences would follow if the soul failed to return quickly enough to reunite with the body, so great care was taken not to rouse people while they slept. As in the western cultures, incubation of dreams was widely practiced in China. Furthermore, images in dreams were thought to have specific meanings. If one dreamed about the sun or moon rising, one's family would prosper. To dream of an orchard loaded with fruit meant that one would have many offspring. Dreaming about teeth falling out signified that one's parents were in danger.

In Africa, dreams have had a long cultural, clinical, and psychospiritual history. Not only the gods, but also as-yet-unborn, living, and dead family members were thought to communicate with the dreamer through dreams. Up to five generations of recently departed ancestors were part of the individual's personal immortality, and connections with the spirit world were made through them.

Native American tribes often believed that dreams were among life's most important experiences. For example, the Iroquois believed that dreams were divinely inspired. Some tribes believed that wishes expressed in dreams needed to be acted out in waking life, so if a dream indicated that the person was giving a feast he would be obligated to provide a feast in waking life. The Mapuche Indians of Chile shared their dreams daily within the family unit, especially in times of physical and emotional stress.

An underlying premise in ancient times generally was that dreams originated outside the dreamer, typically from a higher power. Furthermore, the belief was that the future was fated and could be foretold in dreams. Sleep was thought to be a time when people were freed from worldly constraints and were thus permitted easier access to a higher power. In fact, both Asians and native Americans believed that the soul left the body during sleep, wandering in different places and communicating with gods and other spirits. The ancients were all profoundly convinced of the significance of dreams. Dream interpretation influenced the most serious of all personal, political, and economic decisions. The ancients developed methods to distinguish good from evil dreams, rituals for preparing dreamers to receive good dreams as well as rituals to ward off evil dreaming, dictionaries for interpreting dream symbols, and designations of who could interpret dreams.

0–1900 A.D.

Throughout the time period of 0–1900 A.D., people in several parts of the world maintained their positive views of dreams. For example, dreams have always been important in the Islamic world. Muhammad apparently drew his inspiration for developing the Moslem religion and for his military conquests from his dreams. Although the Muslims were influenced by the Greeks, they did not generally use dreams to diagnose or treat medical problems. Rather than incubating dreams, Muslims sought dreams by reciting prayers during the day.

The Greek Orthodox branch of Christianity continued to value dreams. The writings of Synesius, a fifth-century bishop, sound much like modern thinking about dream interpretation. He thought that dreams were an inexhaustible source of riches, allowing the mind to go to many levels. According to Synesius, dreams could be imaginative, prophetic, and problem solving, but he thought that dream books were of little help in understanding the dreams of a specific individual.

Dreams and dream interpretations were often valued highly by early Western Christian church founders. In the third century, Tertullian wrote that dreams were gifts from God, but that people were not accountable for feelings and actions in their dreams.

Around 300–400 A.D., however, attitudes toward dreams changed in Europe due in large part to the influence of a few people. A wealthy man named Jerome felt quite conflicted between his fondness for pagan classics and his studies of the Bible. He apparently had a dream in which he was dragged before the judgment seat and asked his identity. He replied that he was a Christian but was told he was a liar because he followed Cicero instead of Christ. He was ordered to be scourged. He called out for mercy and took an oath never to possess worldly books again. After this dream, he became a great Bible scholar and consultant. He was called to Rome to translate the entire Hebrew Bible into Latin (later called the Vulgate). In translating the Bible into the Vulgate, Jerome apparently deliberately mistranslated the Hebrew word for witchcraft, "anan," as "observing dreams." Of the 10 times the word "anan" appeared, he translated it correctly 7 times as condemning witchcraft and mistranslated it 3 times. Jerome's mistranslation heralded an end to the rich respect for dreams in the Western culture and changed Christian beliefs and practices for the next 15 centuries. Dream interpretation changed from a spiritual activity to a superstitious one in the eyes of the Catholic Church during this time. At about the same time, Macrobius wrote about nightmares in which demons (incubus and succubus) possessed people sexually during dreams, which further fueled the paranoia about evil spirits.

Around the 11th century, Thomas Aquinas issued warnings about demons in dreams, and thereafter European Christians apparently became obsessed with demons and devils. Dreams were the hunting grounds of the inquisitors. Needless to say, not many people during these times were willing to reveal their dreams, and many tried to suppress having dreams. The medieval Catholic Church further emphasized the prohibition against dreams by suggesting that dreams were not from God and must be ignored. The Church's position was that the word of God was given to the Church, and hence ordinary people did not need God to speak to them through dreams.

After the Middle Ages, the philosophical and scientific community began to rethink dreams, dissociating them from demons and devils and associating them with scientific inquiry. Scientists began to emphasize the physical or somatic features of dreams. For example, Locke, in 1690, proposed that dreams were determined by sensory inputs. In the first American psychiatry book written in 1812, Rush considered dreams as a transient paroxysm of delirium, arising from changes in cerebral blood flow, signifying imperfect sleep and often indicating an impending illness. Wundt, who founded the world's first psychological laboratory in Germany, held that dreams arose mainly from sensory stimuli.

Several individuals began to do self-observations and scientific experiments on the effects of external stimulation on dreams (e.g., Maury and Saint-Denis in France). Several people wrote about dreams during the 19th century. For example, in 1865 Seafield wrote an extensive treatise on dreams in which he stated that dreams were intelligible, reflected the dreamer's personality, could be compensatory, were capable of problem solving, and led to a better-balanced personality if interpreted. Thus, contrary to the popular belief that Freud stimulated the modern interest in dreams, there was growing acceptance of dreaming by scholars in the late 19th century.

EARLY PSYCHOANALYTIC THEORIES
OF DREAM INTERPRETATION

Most of the major "depth psychologists" of the 20th century have attributed great significance to dreams. Indeed, the views of the early psychoanalytic theorists (Freud, Jung, Adler) have had a profound impact on the current view of dreams and dream interpretation; hence, I will review these theories in some detail here.

Sigmund Freud's Theory
of Dream Interpretation

In 1900, Freud wrote the *Interpretation of Dreams,* which he viewed as his most important work. Indeed, Freud's work was very influential in changing the predominant view that dreams are caused by external sources such as gods or demons or by physiological processes to the view that dreams are generated as a result of intrapsychic conflicts. Much of what Freud postulated about the mechanisms of dreams has since been disproven in empirical research, but he has had an enormous impact in restimulating interest in dreams.

Freud believed that dreams have a dual purpose of preserving sleep and acting as a safety valve for unacceptable wishes. He believed that some dreams were stimulated by external and internal stimuli (e.g., an alarm clock, thirst). However, he thought that dreams arose primarily for the fulfillment of our primitive, infantile intrapsychic wishes such as Oedipal longings for the parent of the opposite sex. He believed that occurrences during the day (what he called "day residue") stimulated these infantile wishes. These infantile wishes are not acceptable to our conscious minds and are repressed during waking life when we have more control, but they come out in dreams (usually in distorted forms) because we are not able to censor these thoughts as much during sleep. We need sleep, so the mind compromises by not being quite as vigilant and allowing the distorted versions to slip through. During sleep we do not have to obey either the laws of reality or our superego promises to be good. We dream about our deepest wishes, which allows the repressed parts of ourselves some gratification. Freud felt that our unconscious minds fool us with the imaginary fulfillment of our most strongly felt longings. For Freud, dreams could thus be viewed as a compromise between the need for sleep and the need for the expression of the unresolved memories and impulses.

Freud thought that an examination of these repressed, distorted wishes could help us understand our unresolved urges, hence the notion that dreams are the "royal road to a knowledge of the unconscious activities of the mind" (Freud, 1900/1966, p. 647). According to Freud, an understanding of the different types of distortions is necessary as a stepping stone for dream interpretation, in which one essentially tries to reverse the process of distortion to make the latent content (the underlying meaning) manifest (out in the open). Freudians discuss five types of distortion: condensation (a combination of several images), displacement (one image takes the place of another), secondary elaboration (the dream content is revised as it is recalled to disguise the underlying meaning), dramatization (the presentation of thoughts in a dramatic, exaggerated form), and symbolism (an image in the dream stands for something else).

Freud compared the psychoanalyst doing dream interpretation to an archaeologist uncovering layer after layer of the psyche before coming to the deepest, most valuable treasures. He felt that dreams provide pieces of memory leading to the discovery of the historical problems that perpetuate current emotional difficulties. To get to the latent meaning, Freud said that we must decode the symbols in the dream by examining the thoughts, memories, and feelings that get stirred up by the dream. Obviously, from a Freudian perspective, interpreting one's own dreams would be extremely difficult, if not impossible, because the conscious mind cannot tolerate the expression of infantile wishes.

The primary Freudian method of dream interpretation is free association, in which the dreamer is asked to say whatever comes to mind with as much honesty as possible. Through associations, Freud believed that the dreamer would come to the origins of the conflicts revealed in the dream. Freud listened to the dreams and associations and interpreted them by listening to their rhythm and pattern, comparing them to other thoughts and feelings that the dreamer had expressed. He also used his own associations, as well as his understanding of transference and resistance, in making his interpretations (Schwartz, 1990).

Freud (1900/1966) indicated that only the dreamer had the key to the meaning of the dream. However, he suggested that if the personal level of associations was not revealing, a symbolic interpretation might be needed given that he postulated a form of shared unconscious among all people. Hence, when individual associations failed to yield fruitful results, he thought that the images could represent unconscious universal symbols. He had a list of common symbols that could be used to interpret dream images. Given the sexual emphasis of Freudian theory, most of the symbolism was sexual in nature. For example, long and pointed objects generally were considered to be phallic objects, whereas rounded objects, boxes, and caves were considered to be female objects. Kings and queens were thought to be symbolic of parents. Furthermore, many dreams was considered to reflect Oedipal issues, with men fearing castration and women expressing penis envy.

Freud's contribution to dream interpretation has been incredible, particularly in stimulating interest and acceptance of dreams. No discussion of dreams is complete without a focus on Freud. Beyond the heuristic value, however, perhaps the most lasting contribution has been the discovery of the method of free association, which allows for the personal exploration of the meaning of the dream. On the negative side, evidence has not been found for his claims that dreams represent wish fulfillment, that dreams reflect distorted unconscious issues, or that elements in dreams have universal symbolic meanings. Perhaps the major problem, however, is that exploring dreams from a Freudian perspective can lead to interminable analysis with little immediate application to waking life.

Carl Jung's Theory of Dream Interpretation

Unlike Freud, Jung (1964, 1974) viewed dreams as a normal, creative expression of the unconscious. He thought that dreams served a compensatory function, representing sides of one's personality that could not be allowed in waking life, and that they presented inner truths not yet known to or trusted by conscious awareness. Dreams are thus a key to uniting the conscious and unconscious by helping dreamers become aware of these hidden feelings. Jung rejected Freud's disguise theory and focused on the manifest content of the dream to see what it revealed, rather than what it concealed, about the person's feelings regarding his or her current life. Jung also rejected Freud's reduction of all symbols to a particular idea, postulating instead that some symbols were unique to the individual and others were universal and derived from archetypes in the collective unconscious (shared by all people).

In Jungian therapy, dream interpretation is one of the main treatment methods, with some Jungian therapists (e.g., Bosnak, 1988; Von Franz, 1987, 1988, 1991) using dream interpretation as the sole method of treatment. Jung believed that dreams should be interpreted in whatever way dreamers find most useful. As with Freud, associations were a primary technique to uncover the message of the dream. His method of association differed from Freud's, however, in that Jung wanted to keep the associations as closely connected to the dream image as possible rather than allowing the type of chain associations that Freud used that can depart from the dream image (to be discussed in more detail later). Jung also encouraged dreamers to represent dream images in various forms of artistic expression, including acting out various images in the dream through art, dancing, and music.

As with Freud, Jung believed that the personal level of interpretation, based on the personal unconscious, should be attempted first. If the personal level is not revealing, he suggested interpreting the dream symbols from the level of the collective unconscious because he noted that people across many different cultures share similar dream images. Thus, he would use myths, fables, medieval alchemy, and archetypes to help the dreamer elaborate upon the dream. He called the personal dreams "little dreams," whereas archetypal dreams were sometimes considered "big dreams" because they might have broad implications for more people than the individual person.

Jung's particular contribution regarding dreams was the belief that dreams are positive, normal, and creative, and can be used to help people achieve a balance in waking life. Although there are many aspects of Jungian dream interpretation that I value, I personally have a more difficult time with the emphasis on symbolism, the collective unconscious, and archetypes.

Alfred Adler's Theory of Dream Interpretation

Adler (1936, 1938, 1958) believed that dreams function to preserve the unity of one's personality and sense of self-worth. He viewed dreams as a means for the ego to achieve reassurance, security, and protection against any damage to self-esteem. For Adler, dreams are purposeful and congruent with the lifestyle of the dreamer. He felt that dreams were second only to earliest childhood memories as trustworthy approaches for exploring personality. Rather than viewing dreams as being different from waking thoughts, Adler felt that both were means of rehearsing for future activities and achievements. Indeed, Adler did not mind if a patient made up dreams rather than brought in actual dreams because he considered imagination to be an expression of the patient's style of life. Adlerian therapists focus on the total experience of the dreamer rather than the unconscious strivings, using dreams to discover the client's private logic, biases, and errors in thinking (Krippner, 1990b). Hence, Adler saw the dream as the "royal road to consciousness" (Gold, 1959).

Adler considered dreaming to be an attempt to solve problems and to provide guidance for the future (Ansbacher & Ansbacher, 1956). He thought that dreams served as a bridge connecting the dreamer's problem with his or her goal, a means of rehearsing solutions, and a preparation for attaining the goal. He postulated that people draw emotional strength from dreams to solve their problems. Thus, dreams pave the way for problem solving by reducing a problem to a metaphorical form that can be solved more readily than when we face the problem in waking life.

Adler (1936) also thought that dreams achieve their purpose by employing emotion and mood rather than reason and judgment. Furthermore, he thought that an understanding of a dream was only valid when it could be integrated with the dreamer's general behavior, early memories, and current problems. Of the early analytic thinkers, Adler's notions about dreams are most aligned with the contemporary "continuity theory" of dreaming that dreams are similar to waking thoughts.

Adler was clearly a forerunner of the view that dreams reflect waking life. He presented a refreshing viewpoint that dreams are normal occurrences. Unfortunately, his clinical recommendations for working with dreams are vague. He did not provide clear guidelines for working with dreams in therapy, making if difficult to apply his theory about dream interpretation to practice.

CONTEMPORARY
DREAM INTERPRETATION THEORIES

Despite the emphasis on dream interpretation by the early psychoanalytic theorists, there was a dearth of interest in dream interpretation other than in psychoanalytic circles for much of the middle and latter parts of the 20th century. One could postulate that this lack of interest, at least in the United States, was due to the heavy emphasis on behaviorism and a corresponding lack of interest in internal phenomena (see Hill & Corbett, 1993). Erikson (1954) suggested that dreams went out of fashion in psychiatry in the 1930s because they did not fit well with the emphasis on speed and practicality in the North American culture. He thought that many therapists felt that it took too long to unravel all the associations for even one dream and thus working with dreams took them too far away from everyday life. Cartwright (1993) additionally postulated that the American love affair with science and the mistrust of anything subjective mitigated against using dreams. She also noted that the newfound ability to control abnormal behavior with drugs and behavioral management programs further caused psychotherapy training programs to discard dream interpretation as archaic.

Cartwright (1993) noted, however, that interest in using dreams in psychotherapy has revived in recent years. She attributed the increased interest to revolutionary discoveries about sleep and dreaming that have been made using new methodologies in sleep laboratories and to the development of sleep disorder clinics that help people with sleep disturbances (see Chapter 2). In addition, interest in internal phenomena has once again become acceptable since the advent of the cognitive revolution around 1970 (see Hill & Corbett, 1993). Indeed, the dramatic growth of the Association for the Study of Dreams attests to the interest in dreams, although dream interpretation still has received minimal empirical attention.

Some academics still seem hesitant about dream interpretation. Many view dream interpretation as being "fringy," similar to parapsychology and New Age therapies. I have received some funny looks from colleagues when I tell them that I am interested in dreams and dream interpretation. Perhaps the dismissive stance of scientists throughout the ages suggesting that dreams are just sensory phenomena and the distrust of dreams by Christians during the Middle Ages still persist. I hope that, with more empirical research, dreams and dream interpretation will assume their rightful place in scientific and applied psychology.

In the next section, I focus on several contemporary approaches that have influenced my own thinking about using dream interpretation in therapy. All represent methods that have been developed by practitioners who do dream interpretation. Kramer et al. (1976) identified three primary assumptions underlying all the current theories: (1) dreams are meaningful, orderly, and non random events; (2) the dreamer's waking life is reflected in the content of the dreams; and (3) dreams fulfill an important, adaptive function in the psychological life of the individual.

Contemporary Psychoanalytic Theory

Contemporary psychoanalytic thought, based on the empirical research about dreams conducted since Freud's time, now holds that the manifest dream content is a direct representation of waking life (Fosshage, 1983, 1987; Garma, 1987; Glucksman & Warner, 1987; Natterson, 1980, 1993; Schwartz, 1990). Thus, rather than dreams presenting a distortion of hidden impulses, dreams are thought to reflect waking issues and to further waking efforts at problem solving and conflict resolution. Sexual and aggressive affects that are stimulated but not effectively managed during the day may be expressed in a dream, not as a means of wish fulfillment, but as a way of momentarily completing the psychological task and restoring psychological organization (Fosshage, 1987). Schwartz (1990) noted, however, that a person's issues have a history leading back to childhood. Thus, even though dream content may be stimulated by current concerns, these concerns are characterized by the dreamer's personality, which had its foundation in childhood.

One similarity between the early and contemporary psychoanalytic theorists is the use of free association as the major therapeutic tool to uncover dreamers' feelings and reactions to the day residue that stimulates dreams. Schwartz (1990) suggested that therapists facilitate the dreamer's attempts at free association, particularly by interpreting resistance and transference. The interpretation of resistance often involves understanding why the dreamer has trouble doing associations. Sometimes analysis of resistance involves talking about how a dream is used to keep the therapist away from other material. The interpretation of transference involves analyzing how the relationship between the therapist and dreamer facilitates the specific associations and resistances that occur. Furthermore, psychoanalytic therapists try to determine why a client tells a dream at a particular time, what else is going on in the dreamer's life that connects to the dream, and what the dream means for the ongoing analysis. Schwartz also contended that, although Freud believed that symbols could be interpreted universally because they were part of a deeply repressed common ancestral heritage, most contemporary analysts believe that symbols are an aspect of a general cognitive ability to create likeness and metaphor. Thus, no one-to-one correspondence is required for interpreting symbols. Dream dictionaries are used only to suggest the culturally common usage of images rather than as a manual that dictates the meaning of a symbol.

Contemporary psychoanalytic theory clearly has much to contribute to our knowledge about dream interpretation, particularly in understanding the dynamics of using dreams in therapy. Contemporary psychoanalytic theorists have corrected many of the problems in Freud's dream interpretation theory. The major strengths of psychoanalytic dream interpretation are the use of free association and the development of insight into the dream. Unfortunately, this approach does not focus enough on emotions. Furthermore, there is a danger that clients might not be able to translate insights into action.

Weiss's Method of Dream Analysis

Weiss (1986) developed an approach to dream interpretation based on Rosenthal's (1980) psychoanalytic model of dream interpretation. Rosenthal suggested that the thoughts, feelings, impressions, and ideas that we do not process during the day come out in our dreams. Dreams are comprised of material that we may not be aware of in waking life. Dreams present us as we really are, rather than as we pretend to be during the day. Dreams allow a channel for positive and creative energies as well as a place to discharge unpleasant and unacceptable feelings. Weiss suggested that to understand the messages in dreams, one must learn dream language, which uses nonverbal pictures and images to represent ideas and feelings. Thus, interpretation consists of translating dream symbols into the unique underlying meanings for each person.

Weiss proposed the following six steps for dream analysis: (1) *define a pattern,* which is accomplished by having the dreamer tell the dream in the third person or talk about the general mood or feeling in the dream, and then relate the pattern to waking life; (2) *find a focal point,* which is typically the least understood part of the dream; (3) *define every symbol and get to-the-point associations,* which is important to determine what the symbols stand for and to relate them to waking life; (4) *rewrite the dream story,* substituting the new meanings for the symbols; (5) *arrive at the dream message,* which is what to do or not do in life; (6) *apply the dream message to one's life,* which is crucial for the dream interpretation to be useful. Weiss argued that the most important part of therapy is what the client does with the self-knowledge gained from the dream interpretation.

Weiss's method of dream interpretation is refreshingly straightforward and easy to learn and use. I recommend it particularly for therapists who are just learning different methods of doing dream interpretation and want to try some different techniques. My negative comments are that the model feels a bit rigid and simplistic for wide use in therapy.

Contemporary Jungian Theorists

Jungian theorists (e.g., Beebe, 1993; Bosnak, 1988; Johnson, 1986) have generally stayed relatively close to Jung's original theory. In his dream groups, Bosnak (1988) has dreamers tell the dream slowly and in the present tense. Group members try to feel the emotions in the dream as the dreamer relates the dream. After the dream, all the group members share their physical reactions to the dreams. The task of the group is to work with the depth of the emotions and bring the feelings to the surface so that they no longer manifest themselves in symptoms. This approach is particularly good for getting into emotions.

I particularly like Johnson's (1986) four-step Jungian approach to dream interpretation. First, *associations* form the foundation for interpreting the dream because associations come from the unconscious in response to the dream images. Associations are always done by returning to the original image rather than by making chain associations. Using chain associations, the therapist allows the dreamer to associate to the next image based only on the last image (e.g., in associating to an oil lamp the person might say "lamp," "light," "day," "summer," "vacation," "beach," "swimming," "sharks"), such that by the end of associating the dreamer may have indeed arrived at some personally relevant complex but it may not be one generated by the dream image. In contrast, in associating to an oil lamp using Jungian methods, the therapist would continually bring the dreamer back to associating to oil lamps (e.g., "Oil lamps were used in the 19th century," "Oil lamps are dirty," "Oil lamps don't light very well," "I remember a picture of my grandmother holding an oil lamp").

Johnson indicated that the "correct" association would "click" for the dreamer. One of the associations would generate a lot of energy, fit with the other symbols in the dream, touch a wounded or hurt part, and/or help the person see something new. He suggested that the way to find the essence of the dream symbol is to "go where the energy is" (p. 56) because every symbol is calculated to rouse us, to wake us up. Another way that Johnson suggests therapists find the associations to dream images is through archetypical application, which means looking in myths, fairy tales, and ancient religious traditions for what symbols might mean to the person.

With an understanding of the images, the second step is to *look for the parts of the inner self that are represented by the images.* Johnson believed that each part of the dream represents a part of our inner self, for example, the anima (the female side of men) or the animus (the masculine side of women). Reowning and reintegrating parts of oneself leads to the development of the self, a key goal of Jungian (and Gestalt) therapy.

Third, *interpretation* puts together all the information from the first two steps into a cohesive whole about the meaning of the dream for the dreamer's life. Johnson viewed the dream as being a message from the unconscious, so he believed that the interpretation is a summary of that message. However, Johnson cautioned that a correct interpretation cannot be obtained without going through the first two steps. He suggested that the interpretation should teach the person something he or she did not know before. He also believed that a correct dream interpretation is not likely to inflate one's ego or be self-congratulatory. He felt that the interpretation should keep the responsibility on the person rather than lay the blame on someone else and should fit into the overall context of the dreamer's life.

Rituals, developed in the fourth step, help make the dream more concrete for the dreamer. Johnson suggests that performing rituals based on the dream has the power to intensify the understanding of the dream and to help the person change habits and attitudes. An example of a ritual would be placing flowers on a grave after a person dreamed about talking with her deceased father. Another example would be painting a picture that depicted a dream image. These actions help the person explore the dream further and keep the images alive.

Johnson's approach is very comprehensive and similar to the one that I have proposed in this book. In fact, I have often required therapists-in-training to read Johnson's book prior to training. My differences with Johnson are that I have a different underlying philosophy, structure the stages of interpretation somewhat differently, and have more options for approaching each of the stages.

Existential/Phenomenological/ Humanistic/Experiential Approaches

A number of closely-related theories of dream interpretation have been proposed, all focused on experiential aspects of dream interpretation. Phenomenologists examine dreams as they are presented in conscious experience (Boss, 1958, 1963, 1977; Craig & Walsh, 1993). Boss (1977) disagreed with Freud's assertion that dreams are produced with the intent of concealing something from the dreamer and with Jung's assertion that dreams intend to reveal something. Rather he believed that dreams are just a historical episode in the life of the dreamer. Thus, rather than looking for the disguised meaning of the dream, the dream is dealt with as an experience in and of itself. The goal of therapy is to return to the dream as a vital, concrete episode of being-in-the-world and allow the dreamer to acknowledge and appreciate the experience. Thus, if a person dreams of her sister dying, it is not necessary to ask who the sister represents metaphorically; rather one deals with how it feels for the dreamer to have her sister die.

Craig and Walsh (1993) presented two stages in the pheno-menological analysis of dreams: explication (the gathering of data or context) and elucidation (the manner of interpreting dream-related data). During explication, the dreamer is asked to describe the parts of the dream more fully. As the dreamer describes different parts, he or she remembers more detail and is able to recall and relive the dream as it was actually experienced. The therapist's job is to listen, observe, and question, but to avoid interpreting or imposing his or her viewpoint. The dreamer's job is to tell everything that he or she knows and is willing to share about his or her dream experience. No attempt is made to uncover day residue or childhood memories, although they may occur to the dreamer naturally.

During elucidation, the therapist helps the dreamer find the mean-ing already in the dream without referring to theoretical concepts or symbols or anything beyond the dream itself. The therapist listens to hear what is said and recognized, what is said but unrecognized, and what is never spoken at all. To get to the meanings, therapists must "bracket" or set aside their beliefs about the dream and listen to the dream itself. Craig and Walsh (1993) indicated that dream images refer to themselves (primary allusions), to the kinds of entities they are (secondary allusions), and to corresponding features in waking life (tertiary allusions). Thus, for a specific dreamer, the image of a dog jumping up and down might refer to an overactive dog, to animals in general, or to a demanding person in one's life.

Perls developed the Gestalt approach to dream interpretation. Perls (1969) and Polster and Polster (1973) rejected the idea of the unconscious and focused on the here and now. Perls believed that all the parts of the dream represent parts of oneself and that these parts need to be put together for the person to become whole, hence his view that dreams are the "royal road to integration." He stated that people needed to reown and integrate these disparate parts of their personalities. Therefore, he directed clients to act out the parts of their dreams so that they could get back into reexperiencing the dream and work with the corresponding emotions and conflicts. Thus, with a dream about a rosebush, the therapist would ask the dreamer to become the rosebush and perhaps have the roses and the thorns carry on a dialogue. Perls did not, however, believe in using the technique of interpretation because he felt it interfered with clients coming to their own awareness and inner experiencing.

Several contemporary dream theorists have been influenced by Perls. Faraday (1972, 1974) particularly emphasized the present orientation of dreams. She postulated that the dream can be interpreted at two different levels. At the *reality* level, she suggested that dreams can make us aware of things that may be going on in our lives that we have somehow overlooked. At the *subjective* level, she suggested that dreams function metaphorically to reveal our subjective feelings and attitudes toward life. Faraday thought that whether or not dreams reveal long-standing conflicts, they always reflect how the conflict is manifested in the dreamer's current situation. Further, she hypothesized that dream images form an individualized picture language that varies for each person from situation to situation. Given the individuality of the picture language, she thought that dreamers must draw upon their individual experiences to understand what something means in a dream. Thus, dreams cannot be interpreted according to predetermined symbols.

Delaney (1991, 1993), who was influenced by both Gestalt and Jungian theory, proposed a dream interviewing method in which she asks the dreamer to define and describe the symbols in the dream to her as if she were someone from another planet. Because people often feel silly explaining things that seem obvious, the interviewer's stance of being from another planet allows the dreamers to say what are typically idiosyncratic associations. Delaney's model has seven steps: telling the dream story, getting an overview of the feelings, eliciting adequate definitions and descriptions of the major images, condensing and recapitulating the descriptions, bridging to waking life, summarizing, reflecting and generating options for action. Delaney was particularly eloquent at describing the nonintrusive role of the interviewer that helps the dreamer come to his or her own understanding of the dream. She emphasized that interviewers should not ask "why" questions and should not tell dreamers the meaning of dreams because these interventions stifle the essential act of individuals processing their internal reactions.

Gendlin (1986) and Mahrer (1990) have both described experiential approaches for helping dreamers reexperience the feelings in their dreams. They contend that when a person can connect with or have a "felt sense" of what he or she experienced in a dream, energy is freed up and the person "knows" what the dream is about. From an experiential perspective, when people cannot allow themselves to experience feelings, they become blocked and cannot progress emotionally. However, when people can experience their feelings, they can stay within the flow of their experiencing and move on to new emerging feelings. The important part of this method is to focus on the bodily sensations and feel the emotions that emerge while pondering the dream. Rather than asking the mind for the cognitive connections, the person examines how his or her body feels at different points in the dream. Mahrer (1990) suggested that therapists help clients reenter dreams at moments of peak feelings, relive dreams more fully and deeply, and continue reexperiencing the feelings until clients reach the point of new experience, which should lead to change in one's inner self. Gendlin and Mahrer both stressed that dreamers learn something new, or get a new "growth-direction," from the dream interpretation if they have focused on the bodily feelings in the dream completely. Examples of growth-directions include speaking up for oneself, letting another person get close, and being able to ask for help.

The existential/phenomenological/humanistic/experiential approaches have much to offer. The focus on the dream experience as an important experience in and of itself regardless of what it means symbolically, the necessity for focusing on the immediate experience while working with the dream, the importance of emotions, and the belief in the client are all major contributions to our understanding of dreams. The common element of these approaches is that exploring dreams is not just a sterile intellectual exercise but is a very intense affective experience. I am not convinced, however, that focusing experientially automatically leads the client to insight and action. I believe that therapists have to be more active to work toward insight and action. At the same time, I believe that therapists need to incorporate the crucial experiential philosophy of working collaboratively with the client to facilitate client growth rather than acting as the expert who knows more than the client.

Cartwright's RISC Therapy

In my opinion, Rosalind Cartwright is doing some of the most exciting and best work in dreams and dream interpretation (summarized in Cartwright, 1977; Cartwright & Lamberg, 1992). She has studied dreams in the sleep laboratory and has examined patterns in dreams across the night for different types of people. Recently, she has focused on the use of dream interpretation for people who are in some type of crisis. She has postulated that people do the emotional homework in their dreams that they are too busy and preoccupied to do during the day; thus if people pay attention to their dreams, they recover more quickly from life stress. On the basis of evidence that people have more vivid dreams when they are in crisis, she has postulated that looking at crisis dreams can be a useful way of helping people examine their reactions to the crisis and figure out what they want to do about their situation. Specifically, she postulates that helping people change their crisis dreams will enable them to get control over their emotions. Thus, to lessen depression and a sense of helplessness, Cartwright suggested that people need to learn to rewrite their dream scripts and improve the endings.

Cartwright's RISC method has four steps. The first step is for a person to *recognize* when he or she is having a bad dream. She suggested that the person should become aware while dreaming that the dream is making him or her feel helpless, guilty, or upset. The second step is for the person to *identify* what it is about the dream that makes him or her feel badly. Thus, the person identifies the parts of the dream that portray him or her as being weak or inadequate. Examining dimensions (i.e., opposing states or qualities, such as safety–danger, trust–mistrust, male–female, defiance–compliance) in dreams is particularly helpful to give dreamers an understanding of the way they organize their world. Third, the person needs to *stop* the bad dream. Cartwright stated that dreamers need to realize that they are in charge and have the power to change what happens in their dreams, which are, after all, their own productions. The fourth step is to *change* the dream dimensions into their opposite, positive sides. She suggests that, at first, people may need to practice changing dream dimensions while awake, but, with practice, people can change the action during their dreams.

Cartwright indicates that people can learn the RISC method in brief therapy, sometimes in as few as eight sessions. Using the sleep laboratory, she wakes people from REM sleep and has them relate their dreams to ensure accuracy of dream recall. The therapy proceeds based on the transcripts that are typed immediately. As treatment progresses, home dream diaries are kept, and the dreamer takes a more active role. The dreamer is an active coinvestigator who seeks to understand the present crisis and distressing early life experiences that the dream is attempting to portray. Becoming active in the process empowers the troubled dreamer to change his or her self-image as being victimized, helpless, or rejected. As the dream character takes control, the dreamer tries out this new-found sense of control in waking life, which leads to improvements in functioning. Thus, the RISC method is a therapeutic technique specially developed to promote psychological healing via the use of dreams.

Cartwright's theory is a wonderful example of how therapists can help clients to feel empowered. This approach is particularly appropriate for working in a crisis-intervention mode with very troubling dreams, but may not be as appropriate for general use within insight-oriented therapy.

Integration of Theories

Although at first glance the theories about dream interpretation seem quite disparate, they can be integrated within a framework of a three-stage model of therapy including exploration (associating to the elements of dreams and experiencing the emotions in dreams), insight (understanding the meaning of dreams), and action (making changes based on the message of dreams). Experiential theories—with their emphasis on self-awareness, the dream being an experience in and of itself, reexperiencing of the affect in dreams, and collaborating with the client to come up with the meaning of the dream—fit quite well into the Exploration Stage. Psychoanalytic theorists (e.g., Freud and Jung) fit into both the Exploration and Insight Stages because of their emphasis on associations to the dream images and helping clients arrive at deeper understanding of the meaning of dreams through interpretation. Several of the theories (e.g., Johnson, Weiss, Cartwright, Delaney) discuss strategies to help clients take action on the basis of what they have learned through the process of working with dreams.

I have integrated elements of all of these theories into the model of dream interpretation delineated in the next section of the book, using a framework of the Exploration, Insight, and Action Stages. Rather than just piecing together parts of other theories, however, I have selected methods that fit with my cognitive–experiential model of dream formation and dream interpretation.

SUMMARY

The attribution for dreaming has changed from the ancient belief that dreams were external and sent from gods or demons to the more current belief that dreams reflect the waking thoughts and conflicts of the individual person. Correspondingly, the methods of interpretation have changed from using dream dictionaries to using personal associations as the beliefs in the origins of dreams have changed from external to internal causes.

Throughout the ages there has been some controversy over whether dreams are purely physiological events that arise from sensory inputs (as has been explicated by Aristotle through Hobson) or whether they represent more psychological or even spiritual phenomena (as has been explicated by Plato through Freud and Jung). If one regards dreams as purely physiological, then interpretation is not necessary.

However, if one views dreams as having a psychological origin and function, then interpretation is desirable and even necessary.

Current theories of dream interpretation range from the Freudian belief that interpretation reveals unconscious, forbidden wishes to the more prevalent current belief that interpretation leads to waking conflicts. Different theories yield different methods of working with dreams ranging from working with associations and symbolism to the intensification of emotions. These theories can be integrated through a three-stage model of exploration, insight, and action, which will be explained more thoroughly in the remainder of this book.

❦

Explication of the Cognitive–Experiential Model of Dream Formation and Dream Interpretation

CHAPTER FOUR

A Cognitive–Experiential Model of Dream Formation and Dream Interpretation

BELIEFS AND ASSUMPTIONS about the origin and function of dreams lay the foundation for one's model of dream interpretation. For example, because Freud (1900/1966) believed that dreams represented disguised unconscious wishes, he formulated an interpretive, symbolic model of dream interpretation that allows therapists to help clients go from the disguised manifest level of dream images to the unconscious latent dream content. In contrast, Perls (1969) rejected the idea of the unconscious and focused on the here and now. He believed that all the parts of the dream represented parts of the self and that people needed to reown these parts of their personalities. Hence, he developed an experiential method of dream interpretation that encouraged dreamers to act out different parts of dreams. Using my understanding of the most recent theory and research on sleep and dreaming (see Chapter 2) and the history of dream interpretation (see Chapter 3), this chapter presents my beliefs about what dreams are and how they are formed. Then using this foundation of a cognitive–experiential model of dream formation, I present an overview of my approach to dream interpretation.

WHAT ARE DREAMS?

Even though our bodies are resting and external stimulation is minimized during sleep, our minds do not stop working. During non-rapid-eye-movement (NREM) sleep, mentation is similar to waking thought patterns, but during rapid-eye-movement (REM) sleep, mentation

47

takes on a different, more creative, more playful quality than daytime thought or NREM mentation. In NREM mentation, we think literally and directly about waking concerns, whereas REM sleep takes on a more imagistic, metaphorical quality in which we create a story about the waking problems.

One way in which REM mentation differs from waking thought or NREM mentation is in the language used in dreams (Kramer, 1993). Dream language is less structured, less connected, and more fluid than waking thought, and it is not to be taken literally (Kramer, Moshiri, & Scharf, 1982). Cartwright and Lamberg (1992) noted that dreams come in pictures rather than words, so that they are like the hieroglyphics of ancient Egypt that need to be decoded on the basis of what is in our memory banks to be understood. The language of dreaming seems to make use of two essentially human communication characteristics: the use of metaphors and our propensity to tell stories.

As humans we tend to conceptualize our world metaphorically. If you listen to people, you will notice metaphors sprinkled throughout speech (e.g., "He's tough as nails," "It rolled off her tongue like honey," or "She built a wall around herself"). Metaphors capture much of our feeling and experience in a graphic characterization of images. Some theories (e.g., Hall, 1953; Lakoff, 1993) place metaphors at the heart of language development and comprehension. Infants probably think in images prior to the development of language, so that much of our early learning may be captured in images rather than words. Images and metaphors thus may form the basis for understanding the meanings of words. In dreams and in waking life, then, we seem to rely on the more elemental images and metaphors to express our underlying feelings. Indeed, metaphors have been found to be particularly useful in therapy as a way for therapists and clients to express underlying feelings (Hill & Regan, 1991; McMullen, 1995).

Furthermore, we seem to be storytelling creatures (Howard, 1991, 1992). Stories and myths are present in all human cultures. Certainly the prevalence of books, movies, and television in our lives indicates that many people in our culture are very engaged by stories. When something happens, we want to tell our stories to other people. The Bible and the Koran teach through parables, perhaps because people react more positively to stories than to direct lecturing. Ericksonian hypnotic therapy (see Haley, 1973) also uses stories and indirect communication to influence people and circumvent defenses. Because stories, like metaphors, involve emotions, morals, images, and ideas, they seem to be more profoundly arousing to us than direct communication.

Perhaps metaphors and stories enable us to remember concepts better than just trying to remember facts because the visual images evoked by metaphors and stories stimulate several of the senses. Current theories suggest that an experience is more likely to be encoded initially into memory if it evokes several of the senses, and memories are more easily retrieved when there are more cues that trigger the memory (Glass & Holyoak, 1986; Medin & Ross, 1992). Thus, during our dreams, we weave stories from thoughts and feelings about ourselves in the present with relevant memories from the past. Actually, we do not just tell ourselves the stories, we enact the stories as if we were in a play or a movie. As Cartwright and Lamberg (1992) stated, we create the script, set up the scene, produce and direct the show, and play the starring role. Snyder (1970) found that the dreamer appears in 95% of his or her dreams and almost always plays a starring role. Thus, dreams are more than simple rehashes of waking events—they are creations that are at different times mundane, fun, adventurous, sexual, wild, crazy, frightening, troubling, or traumatic.

THE ORIGIN OF DREAMS

Although no one is completely sure how dreams come about or what the function of dreaming is, we can speculate on the origin of dreams based on the available evidence from cognitive psychology about thinking and memory (see also Cartwright, 1990; Caspar, Rothenfluh, & Segal, 1992; Epstein, 1994; Glass & Holyoak, 1986; Globus, 1993; Loftus, 1988; Medin & Ross, 1992).

Storage of Memories

Let me take a side excursion to talk about how memories are stored in the brain, because this storage has relevance to dream formation. No one knows for sure how or where all this information is stored in the brain, but we do know that information is distributed across thousands of neurons rather than being stored in single brain cells (Medin & Ross, 1992). Cognitive scientists postulate that information is stored in schemata, which Mahoney (1991) defined as "abstract structures that comprise and/or generate patterns or themes of experience" (p. 78). Schemata are clusters of related thoughts, feelings, sensations, memories, and actions (Cartwright, 1990; Cartwright & Lamberg, 1992; Glass & Holyoak, 1986; L. S. Greenberg, Rice, & Elliott, 1993; Medin & Ross, 1992; Stein, 1992). It is important to note that these schemata are cognitive, affective, and behavioral. Components are intertwined in schemata, and thus one cannot separate the various components or consider them in isolation.

Only those details to which we attend in our waking lives are encoded in our memories, so that events that we do not notice on at least a subliminal level do not get stored in our memories. Encoded events that are particularly salient (i.e., those that involve particularly vivid images and that are thought about a lot) assume the most importance within a schema. Information in a schema, however, is not retained at the same rate. Memories that are brought back into awareness and thought about again remain prominent in the schema, whereas others that are unused fade away. In addition, memories often change or become distorted over time so that what is stored is not always accurate (Loftus, 1988).

Within each schema are individual elements (or what have been labelled nodes or units). Elements within each schema are connected to other elements in the schema and to elements in other schemata through links, such that elements that are closely related for an individual have positive or excitatory connections (e.g., the elements of dreams and nightmares may be closely connected for a person), whereas others that are minimally related or unrelated for an individual have negative or inhibitory connections (e.g., the elements of dreams and trucks may be negatively connected for a person). Furthermore, these connections can change with use or disuse, such that the continual activation of a connection strengthens it, whereas a lack of use weakens the connection. An important point is that when one part of a network is activated, the parts of the network that have positive or excitatory connections are also activated.

As an example, Person A might have a schema for examinations. This schema might involve the following elements: catastrophic thoughts about how awful it would be if he could not handle the exam situation, feelings of anxiety and panic, bodily sensations of heart palpitations and sweaty palms, memories of specific situations in which he was anxious during exams, and specific ways that he typically performs during exams. The examination schema might have positive or excitatory connections with a schema of failure, such that the two schemata share a lot of the same elements (e.g., memories in which the person failed, negative reactions of others to failure, and missed opportunities). Each schema, of course, also has unique elements, such that the examination schema might include various studying strategies whereas the failure schema might include thoughts about how to overcome failure. Whenever Person A thinks about exams, he might often think about failure because of the positive connections between these two schemata.

Of course the schematic networks are unique to each individual. For Person B, the examination schema might have positive connections with achievement and success schemata. Hence, in contrast to Person A, Person B might often think about success and getting ahead when she thinks about taking examinations.

Information is stored (encoded) in one or more schemata, and the schemata are arranged within a network. A connectionist or parallel distributing processing (PDP) model (Caspar et al., 1992; Medin & Ross, 1992; Rummelhart & McClelland, 1986) seems to provide the best current description of the relationships among the schemata within the network. According to this PDP model, firings across the network take place in a parallel manner rather than a sequential manner, allowing for very fast processing of information.

Waking Issues Trigger Schemata

Thus, we can understand people's reactions to waking events as being based on what is stored in their schemata. For example, my experience of being upset by an interaction with a colleague might trigger memories of negative interactions with my sister. I might react to my colleague in the same angry, hostile manner that I reacted to my sister in similar situations during childhood fights. Later, I might wonder why I had such an immediate, seemingly irrational, reaction to my colleague's relatively innocuous comment. I might not have "consciously" recognized the connection between my reaction to my colleague and fights with my sister. The associations happen rapidly and are not always logically sequenced because of the rapid connections within the model. We do not usually take the time to trace back through all the connections to figure out why the associations occurred.

A great deal of evidence indicates that dreams often are triggered by events or issues that are salient to us during waking life (see Breger, 1967, 1969; Cartwright, 1990; Garma, 1987; R. Greenberg, 1987; Koulack, 1991; Kramer, 1982; Kramer et al., 1976). During our waking lives, we are bombarded with both external and internal stimuli. We interact with people; we see a wealth of environmental stimuli; we are required to do many tasks. These events are not just external happenings, but can also be emotions, anticipations of future events, or existential concerns and anxieties. When events occur, we react on the basis of the memories of past experiences stored in our brains about that stimulus.

Sometimes our immediate experience is congruent with what is in our schemata, and the situation passes without much impact. At other times our immediate experience is discrepant with what is stored in our schemata. This situation may lead to distress because there is no way to understand the experience. It does not fit with past experiences stored in our schemata. Either we accommodate by changing our schemata to incorporate this new experience (e.g., change our way of thinking to handle new information), or we change the experience to fit into our schemata (e.g., distort or deny experiences so that we do not have to change our schemata). For example, some people have a hard time handling feelings of anger because they have been taught as children to try to make everybody happy. If someone makes them mad, they might not allow themselves to have the feelings. But at an experiential level, they might still be enraged. Discrepancies between experience and self-concept (or what could be called self-schemata) are at the core of much of what we consider to be psychological disturbance (see Kelly, 1955; Rogers, 1942, 1951).

Another important issue is that during the day, many internal and external stimuli impinge upon us. We cannot attend to or respond to all of these things consciously, but they may still have an impact on us at some subconscious level. We may have attended to these things on the periphery of awareness so that they do get encoded into memories. For example, a friend might frown at me during the day but I do not think about it at the time or perhaps I cannot allow myself to feel upset at the time, but the feelings might persist at another level.

As different schemata are activated, less activation is available for previously activated schemata. These previously activated schemata are probably "turned off" unless they are positively connected with the newly activated schemata. Thus, at the end of the day, not all schemata are activated—just those that are particularly salient and "turned on."

The important issue here is that we react to internal and external events that occur during the day based on our past experiences. We do not come to new experiences with a "tabula rasa," but filter our perceptions through thoughts, feelings, and memories stored in our schemata. Hence, people react differently to the same situation because they have different memories. Furthermore, the events that occur during the day cause specific cognitive schemata to be aroused or activated. This state of arousal persists when we go to sleep as we try to make sense of things that happened during the day. Thus, when we go to sleep, we are left with many unfinished feelings and issues from the day. In other words, various schemata are in a state of activation when we go to sleep.

Activated Schemata Stimulate Dreams

When we go to sleep, some schemata are still aroused. Although many urges, feelings, and meanings have occurred to us during the day, not all of them are still salient when we go to sleep. The ones that are salient are probably those that had to do with unrequited urges, unresolved feelings and issues, and highly significant meanings (even if the meanings are out of awareness). Thus, when we go to sleep, we think about problems during NREM sleep much as we do during waking thought and we dream (make stories) about them in REM sleep. Thus, we dream about the issues that concerned us most, gave us the most pleasure, or stimulated us most during the day. Without much external stimulation, we keep processing the internal stimulation (i.e., our memories). Our dreams thus appear to be a mechanism by which we try to process the salient information and emotions that have occurred to us and attempt to fit them into the appropriate schemata. Too much happens during the day to be able to deal with all of it, so we sort it out at night during our dreams. In this way, dreams seem to afford us the opportunity to work through emotions and problems that occur during waking life.

The stimuli that trigger dreams can range from the trivial to the profound. However, it is important to note that what seems trivial to one person might be profound to another. A parking ticket might be inconsequential to one person but send another person into a deep depression. Furthermore, the triggering events are not always meaningful in and of themselves but can stimulate past memories that are laden with meaning. One client told me that her dream was just a repeat of part of a television show that she had seen the night before. As we explored the dream, it quickly became apparent that she had only incorporated the portion of the television show that was relevant to specific unresolved personal memories. Thus, people probably relate most strongly to those stimuli in waking life that hold personal relevance for them.

The triggering events are not always external; thoughts about past events and anticipations of future events can also trigger schemata (although perhaps the trigger is always external if one searched hard enough to find it). For example, I might look at my schedule for the day, note that I have little free time, and then start panicking about a speech that I have to give in a few months because the speech stimulates schemata of performance and feared humiliation. The speech is so much on my mind that it takes very little to trigger thinking about it. Hence, I might dream about speeches and remembered humiliations. This example illustrates how anticipations of future events can be as provocative as actual experiences. Likewise, the trigger events are not always just from the past day, but can be from the past if the event remains salient in the person's awareness. For example, ruminations about a fight a week ago with a spouse or a remembered event from childhood might be very much on a person's mind when she goes to sleep.

Let me give an example of how the dream formation process works. Perhaps a person felt depressed and angry all day long but could not allow herself to think about the reasons for her unhappiness. At some level though, she knows that her spouse has been inattentive and insensitive, as he often has been in the past. This is a painful issue for her to deal with because if she thinks about it too much she will have to confront her spouse or make some decisions about her life. Instead, she avoids the issue during waking life. Perhaps some other events also happened that day that were salient although not to the degree of the situation with her spouse—she was scared because she almost hit a rabbit that was crossing the road; she thought of her best friend whom she had not seen for some time; and she could not find her favorite white nightgown when she went to bed. She dreams of a ruthless pirate (her husband) coming after her and her best friend.

As they are trying to escape, a white (from the nightgown) rabbit (from the near-accident) runs in front of them and goes down a hole in the ground (from associations with memories of the white rabbit from *Alice in Wonderland*). The dream thus centers around the pirate (because of the pervasiveness of the feelings about her spouse) but other, less salient, miscellaneous events from the day (rabbit, friend) and activated past memories (the story of *Alice in Wonderland*) are also woven into the dream. Hence, the dreamer has not reviewed the whole day in this dream but has integrated a few of the most salient events into one of the night's dreams (recall that there are four to five dreams per night).

The Dream

The dream does not simply piece these fragments of memory together, but rather represents our active attempt to process our experiences in light of how we have processed past experiences. Cartwright and Lamberg (1992) noted that "dreams don't reflect life only as we currently perceive it, but rather as we feel, imagine, and want it to be" (p. 97). The dream thus weaves together a story that integrates the waking events with what is stored in the schemata in an effort to make sense of the waking events. Hence, I might weave together in my dream an event from childhood in which I felt guilty because of a fight I had with my sister with the current situation of the dispute with my colleague. In my dream, my sister might be running to the department chair to tell him that I should be punished for breaking her favorite doll. Thus, my dream illustrates that my anxiety over the conflict with my colleague is in part due to the upsets that happened when I got in trouble because of fights with my sister when we were children. I am still trying to figure out how to relate to people who are angry at me.

If, in waking life, a person had an event in which his boss was threatening and hostile, schemata of authority and hostility might be activated. In his dream, the hostile boss might be represented by a tyrannical king who rules his kingdom unfairly and arbitrarily because of a memory of having seen this image many times in books and movies. Or if, in waking life, a person is having a midlife crisis and is pondering whether he has done anything worthwhile in his life, he might dream that St. Peter is asking him to account for his life. The image of St. Peter might be invoked because this was an image used by his religion as a metaphor for accounting for one's life.

We can predict neither which schemata nor which images within the schemata will be activated during dreaming. Dreaming is an idiosyncratic process, the network of schemata is enormous, and events are not necessarily encoded accurately for the time of occurrence.

The metaphoric quality of dreams is probably related to the fact that many of our memories are rich in images. Images often help to summarize the content of schemata, giving credence to the phrase, "A picture is worth a thousand words." For example, during the day I may have felt compelled to be nice at a departmental function and may not be aware of my underlying reactions to the event, but at night I might dream that I am being attacked by vicious tigers in the jungle because tigers represent an image or metaphor for me of aggression. Thus, what dreams seem to do is to take our thoughts, feelings, and images from the recent past and our anticipations about the future and weave them together into a story that helps us process our waking experiences. In this manner, waking experiences come to be assimilated into our schemata so that they become memories.

The connectionist model can be used to explain bizarre associations that occur within dreams. Activation across related schemata sometimes causes elements to be evoked that are not related to each other. Thus, activation of the examination schema might stimulate a memory in the failure schema (e.g., the failure of a bank during the depression) that seems irrelevant to the immediate situation.

Successful Dreams

When we are at peace with ourselves and the world, we tend to sleep soundly and dream regularly but remember few of our dreams (Cartwright & Lamberg, 1992). Thus, if nothing particularly troubling has happened recently, if recent events do not trigger troubling memories, or if we do not have major unresolved problems that demand attention, our dreams do not appear particularly troubling. We are more free to play in our dreams, to have adventures or sexual fantasies, or to be creative. Many examples have been cited of people creating artwork, plays, movies, books, scientific discoveries, and technological breakthroughs in dreams (Van de Castle, 1994). In our dreams we do many of the same things we do during daytime thought and fantasy but with perhaps more abandon and fun because we tend not to limit our options as much. When something positive is lacking in our waking lives, our dreams sometimes compensate. One example of this from my own life is that when I have not had much opportunity to do escape reading (something I love to do), I compensate by making up my own adventures in my dreams.

Thus, when we are not under stress, our dreams seem to help us sort our current emotional experiences, compare these to memories, and think ahead to plan our futures. Cartwright and Lamberg (1992) suggested that the dream system is self-regulatory, functioning smoothly to integrate new information when life is calm.

Graphically, the process of successful dreams in helping to assimilate events into schemata is shown in Figure 4.1.

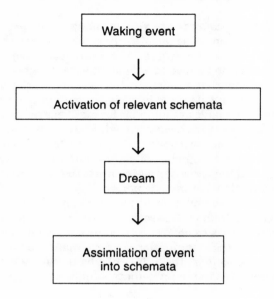

FIGURE 4.1. A graphic representation of how successful dreams operate to assimilate waking events in schemata.

Failure of Dreams to Assimilate Waking Issues

When we are worried, have a bad conscience, or are excited by strong feelings before sleep, we sleep more lightly. Often we remember our dreams more during these times. Cartwright and Lamberg (1992) suggested that intense emotions and light sleep seem to facilitate dream recall because we wake before the dream is over, making it easier to recall the dream.

Generally, the more salient or troubling the waking issues, the more vivid and salient the dreams will probably be, although we seem to be able to divert ourselves from thinking about crucial issues even in our dreams (Cartwright & Lamberg, 1992). We typically remember the most salient dreams, although there are clear individual differences, with some people being more able than others to remember their dreams (see Chapter 2).

The more helpless we feel during the day, the more fear is left over for dreaming to handle at night. Hartmann (1984) found that almost everyone experiencing a traumatic event had dreams and nightmares about it for weeks after the event. The more severe the trauma, the greater the impact on sleep and dreams. Of course, it is important to keep in mind that the perception of severity is highly individual.

Putnam (1989) suggested that some people segregate affectively laden material, such as sexual abuse, in their memory such that it is stored in memory but is not connected with the network of schemata. He speculated that because this affectively laden material is segregated from regular memory, it is not subject to the same triggers that normal memories are subject to. In effect, he suggested that these are state-dependent memories, which are not recalled unless there are very specific triggers, such as particular smells that occurred during the trauma. Thus, some memories may be segregated from other memories because they are too painful.

The phenomenon of stressful dreams is illustrated most clearly in posttraumatic stress disorder (PTSD) dreams, where dreamers dream of the traumatic event over and over again, often waking in fright. It is as if the dream mechanism is stuck because of the overwhelming nature of the trauma (Cartwright & Lamberg, 1992; Hartmann, 1984). In such cases, the PTSD victim cannot internalize the experience into his or her self-concept because there are simply no schemata for such an event. For example, most of us simply cannot comprehend atrocities such as those that occurred during the Holocaust and the Vietnam War. We have no schemata for such horror; rather, we think of the world as a just and fair place. Hence, there is no place for this experience to fit in our schemata.

In contrast to PTSD dreams, recurrent dreams seem to represent a slightly less overwhelming amount of trauma. Rather than being exact replicas of the traumatic event as PTSD dreams are, they weave the stressful issue into a theme that recurs across dreams. The exact rendition of the theme changes in accord with the person's current attempts to deal with the chronic situation. Recurrent dreams seem to reflect ongoing unresolved conflict (Domhoff, 1993). As with nightmares, the dream seems to be unable to cope with processing and assimilating the information and emotions into the existing schemata. Fortunately, clinical evidence suggests that recurrent dreams and nightmares often disappear when precipitating problems are resolved, although some evidence suggests that the nightmares recur when people experience another stressful event (Cartwright, 1979; Hartmann, 1984).

Sleep terrors are another form of stressful dream (Cartwright, 1993; Cartwright & Lamberg, 1992). People who have sleep terrors often seem to function adequately during the day, but are overcontrolled and hostile. They have often experienced a major stressful event in which they felt powerless and impotent. Interestingly, they tend to have minimal amounts of REM sleep, so they do not dream out their affective problems. Instead, they arouse abruptly from deep sleep (NREM sleep) often during the first hour of sleep with a scream and confusion, often engaging in violent acts. Cartwright (1993) speculated that the affect that normally triggers the search for similarly toned, emotionally related memories during REM sleep instead explodes into immediate action often with disastrous consequences. The affect state is expressed without the associated memories of previous solutions to similar problems that might help the person resolve the problem.

Thus, recurrent dreams, nightmares, and sleep terrors are all examples of the inability of the dream function to assimilate events into existing schemata, typically either because no relevant schemata exist or because the experiences are so discrepant from existing schemata. The graphic representation of this process is shown in Figure 4.2.

Summary of Dream Formation

In sum, dreams seem to help us understand what has happened to us during our waking life. They help us process the overwhelming amount of information and emotions that occur during waking life by comparing them to past solutions. Memories are encoded or assimilated into the appropriate schemata when we dream about them. Under stress, however, the dreams seem not to be able to fulfill their function as readily and we have recurrent dreams, nightmares, or sleep terrors.

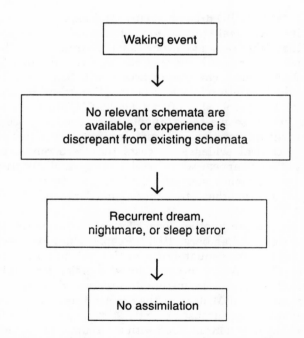

FIGURE 4.2. A graphic representation of the formation of recurrent dreams, nightmares, and sleep terrors.

UNDERSTANDING DREAMS

Although dreams seem to help people encode or assimilate their waking experiences into the appropriate schemata, they probably have minimal impact on changing or restructuring schemata (accommodation). There is a fundamental difference between assimilation and accommodation (Piaget, 1962, 1970; Stiles et al., 1990). With assimilation, things are incorporated into existing schemata. In accommodation, the schemata themselves have to change to be able to incorporate new information.

Thus, mundane dreams, as Hunt (1989) called them, might not really need to be remembered and worked on because they are doing the maintenance work of fitting experiences into available schemata. Of course, it can be valuable to work on these dreams in the sense that you can always learn something new about yourself, but it is probably not imperative to work with these dreams in therapy. On the other hand, some types of dreams do seem to require attention in therapy: particularly vivid or salient dreams, troubling dreams, recurrent dreams, nightmares, or sleep terrors. These types of dreams all seem to reflect issues that need to be dealt with. These dreams seem to occur because the existing schemata cannot assimilate an experience; they signal that the existing schemata need to be restructured to be able to accommodate new data.

Similarly, Breger et al. (1971) suggested that dreams have minimal immediate impact on subsequent waking behavior unless the dreams are understood and worked on. In this view, dreams have meaning and function but exert no effect on postsleep states or traits without further integrative work (Cartwright, 1990). Thus, dreams set the stage or provide us with raw material, but we need to work on what the dream means to us to reap the full beneficial effect of changes in our schematic structures. From a cognitive–experiential perspective, this view suggests that schemata themselves remain unchanged structurally unless the dream is used to help the person integrate new understanding during waking life. By working with our dreams, we can learn about the reasons for our reactions to situations in waking life.

The goal of dream interpretation is to reactivate and change the relevant schemata so that they become more open and able to assimilate experiences. It appears that schemata need to be activated in an emotionally arousing way before they are open to revision (L. S. Greenberg et al., 1993). I propose that the relevant schemata can be activated through the use of associations and reexperiencing the affect of a dream. By exploring the content of the relevant schemata during therapy, we continue the process that the person started during dreaming of trying to figure out how current experiences relate to past experiences. Obviously, given that dreams are triggered by the person's waking events and are associated with material in his or her schemata, the individual is the only person who can provide the meaning of the dream. Dream dictionaries cannot reflect the content of an individual's schemata, although they may be accurate representations of cultural norms of the society in which the person lives.

Through exploration of schemata, people come to greater understanding of themselves. Such understanding can result in altered schematic structures, whereby existing schemata actually change or accommodate to accept new ways of storing information. For example, a woman who previously felt guilty about expressing anger might be able to unravel her issues about being expressive. Through analyzing her dream about going on a shooting spree, she might come to understand that she feels guilty because her mother got angry and abusive whenever she expressed anything other than total compliance. Her therapist might teach her that it is okay to express anger openly in an appropriate manner and encourage her to express anger in the therapeutic relationship. If she accepts them, the therapist's teachings can cause her schemata to accommodate (reorganize). The link between the expression of anger and guilt is weakened (although probably never eradicated), whereas the link between the appropriate expression of anger and the expectation of positive reactions from others is strengthened. If the woman tries the new behaviors and gets positive responses from her therapist and friends, the positive connections are strengthened. Further practice with the new behaviors is obviously necessary to strengthen the new connections and weaken the old connections.

Under periods of stress, however, old connections might reassert themselves and thus be reinforced. Presumably, when we are under stress, we fall back on deeply ingrained coping strategies because newer strategies may fail to lower stress or because increased stress is a very powerful cue for activating older coping strategies. Thus, if someone is negative to this woman when she becomes angry, she might become frightened again as she did when she was a child and revert to compliant, unassertive behavior.

Hence, in dream interpretation we reverse the dream formation process and use the dream as a mechanism for exploring the relevant schemata to uncover the memories that cause the person to react as he or she does to current events in waking life. Furthermore, thorough exploration of the schemata can lead to greater understanding and, hence, to a change in the schematic structure. As a person puts thoughts, feelings, and memories together in a new way, the schemata are rearranged in new patterns, which facilitates greater cognitive flexibility and mental health.

Although the process of interpretation involves exploring schematic structures, therapists do not need to identify which specific schematic structures are involved. Schemata relate to the way the information is organized within the mind. The important issue is not which specific schemata are activated; rather the important issue is the specific thoughts, feelings, and memories that are contained within the schemata. The discussion about schemata is crucial only to explain the process of dream formation and dream interpretation. The process of dream interpretation is shown graphically in Figure 4.3.

One could argue that schemata could be reorganized without dream interpretation. I would agree with this argument because I think this model is a good representation of what we do all the time, particularly in therapy. One of the most typical interventions in therapy is to take a recent event and try to understand why the client reacts as he

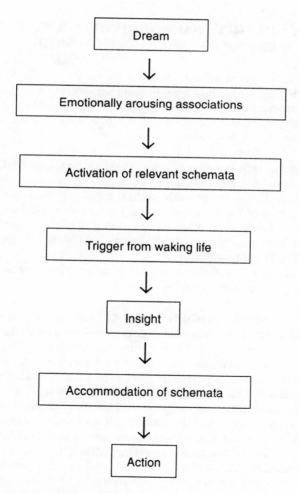

FIGURE 4.3. The model of dream interpretation, moving from the dream images to understanding and action.

or she does in light of previous experiences. I would postulate, however, that dreams are especially helpful in this regard because they use images, metaphors, and stories that are idiosyncratic and provide a window into the person's way of constructing his or her reality. Dream interpretation also sometimes points the way to connections and memories that we have a difficult time accessing via direct communication. Dreams often provide graphic illustrations of our difficulties in living. Furthermore, I would repeat that when clients bring in troubling dreams, these need to be dealt with in therapy so that clients can understand more about the source of the dreams and about themselves.

THEORETICAL BACKGROUND FOR THE HILL DREAM INTERPRETATION MODEL

In choosing a way to work with dreams, we need to pick techniques that allow us to activate, explore, and change the schemata. The model of dream interpretation that I propose draws from several existing models but has integrated the components in a new way. The model is based on the following assumptions:

- Dreams reflect waking rather than unconscious conflicts.
- Dreams are personal and hence cannot be interpreted with a dream dictionary or with standard symbolic interpretations.
- The role of the therapist is as a guide and collaborator rather than an expert who knows the meaning of the dream.
- The best way to work with dreams involves both cognitive and affective components.
- Exploration, insight, and action are all necessary steps of a complete dream interpretation.

I propose a model in which therapists first help clients to associate in an emotionally arousing manner. Associations allow the dreamer to gain access to the schemata to figure out the connections between waking events and memories. The emotional arousal seems to be necessary to enable the schemata to become fully activated and open to change. Once the relevant schemata are activated fully, they can be changed through new understandings and insights. By putting things together in new ways, the schemata begin to change. Once new connections have been made, behavioral changes reinforce the changes in the schemata. Acting on the new connections strengthens them and makes them more stable. These stages flow naturally, with knowledge derived from exploration used to develop the understanding of the dream, and action flowing from the new understanding.

The three-stage model (Exploration, Insight, Action) for dream interpretation is similar to the three-stage models proposed by Carkhuff (1969) and Egan (1986) for therapy. In the *Exploration Stage* of dream interpretation, therapists take a client-centered stance to help clients experientially focus on feelings and cognitions in associating to dream images and linking these images to waking life. The goal of the Exploration Stage is to help clients think of different possible feelings and meanings for each of the pieces of the dream. In the *Insight Stage,* therapists use what they learned about clients in the Exploration Stage as well as their own perspectives to help clients come to some new understandings about themselves. Through collaboration, they try to come to some determination of the meaning of the dream, fitting all the pieces of the dream together. In the *Action Stage,* therapists help clients figure out what to do differently in their lives based on what they have learned throughout the Exploration and Insight stages. The goal of this stage is to help clients incorporate what they have learned by acting on it in waking life. During the latter two stages, therapists often cycle back through earlier stages as new material arises.

The therapeutic relationship and collaboration with the client is essential in all stages. Therapists are facilitators rather than experts in that they help clients come to some personal understanding of the meaning of the dream, help to restructure the schemata, and guide the client in choosing desired actions. The three stages are presented in detail in the Chapters 5–7, with therapeutic issues that arise in using the model presented in Chapter 8. Examples of using the dream interpretation model are presented throughout Chapters 5–7 and in Chapters 9–11.

CHAPTER FIVE

Exploration Stage

T HE EXPLORATION STAGE is the most important stage in the model because exploration allows clients to reexperience their feelings from the dream and expand on these feelings cognitively to figure out how the dream relates to waking events and memories (see Chapter 4). This chapter presents the theory behind the Exploration Stage and provides guidelines for how to implement the stage. Throughout the chapter, brief examples of techniques are presented to illustrate how therapists can help clients explore their dreams. At the end of the chapter, an extended example of a therapist implementing this stage with a client is presented. Table 5.1 shows the goals of the stage, the tasks to be accomplished, the most frequently used and rarely used therapist techniques, and the desired therapist manner in implementing the stage.

PRELIMINARY ISSUES

For the purposes of describing the model, I will assume that a client has brought a dream into therapy that is particularly salient and has asked his or her therapist for help in trying to understand it. Suggestions about how to encourage clients to bring dreams in to therapy and how to deal with therapeutic issues that arise in using the model are presented in Chapter 8.

Generally, therapists will work with just one dream during a given session and will spend at least one whole session on the dream. Trying to understand more than one dream is difficult because of all the complexities of each dream and the limitations of time. The client could present just a fragment of a dream, however, as valuable information can be gained from any portion of a dream.

As the client retells the dream, the therapist will probably want to write down the main images, perhaps using a format such as is shown in Figure 5.1 after the extended example at the end of the chapter. Dreams are often very complicated and illogical, making it difficult even for therapists with great memories to remember details. By jotting down the images as clients talk, therapists can refer back to the specific images during the later steps of the model. Although difficult, it is of course important to maintain eye contact while writing down the images. It is also important to allow the client to tell the dream at his or her own pace to facilitate reentry into the dream. Hence, therapists need to juggle maintaining rapport with getting the key images down on paper.

TABLE 5.1. Outline for Exploration Stage

I. Goals
  A. Learn more about the dream.
  B. Facilitate client reimmersion into the experience of the dream.
  C. Build and/or maintain therapeutic alliance.

II. Tasks
  A. Ask client to retell the dream in the present tense.
  B. Ask how client felt about the dream.
  C. Associate to dream images.
    1. Go through the major images sequentially.
    2. Keep coming back to the specific image.
    3. Do steps of association:
      a. Describe dream images.
      b. Associate to images.
  D. Evoke emotional arousal (optional).
    1. Reflect and intensify feelings.
    2. Be the image.
  E. Link associations of images to waking life to find the trigger of the dream.
  F. Work with conflicts (optional).

III. Therapist techniques
  A. Frequently used techniques: Open-ended questions, reflection of feelings, minimal encouragers, nonverbal encouragers, offering associations "as if it were my dream"
  B. Rarely used techniques: Interpretation, confrontation, direct guidance, information

IV. Therapist manner
  A. Collaborative
  B. Facilitative
  C. Nonintrusive

RETELLING THE DREAM

I generally ask the dreamer to retell the dream in the present tense as if he or she were experiencing it in the immediate moment (see also Enright, 1970). For example, rather than

I dreamed about rats last night.

or

I was walking down this muddy street with rats all around. I went into a building that seemed like a warehouse. It was dark and there were little rustling sounds all around. I heard a cat prowling around and there was a loud crash. Then I was riding across a pond in a horse-drawn sleigh. I'm not sure where we were going, but we were going fast.

I would ask the client to use the present tense as follows:

I am walking down this muddy street with rats all around. I'm a little anxious. I go into a building that seems like a warehouse. It's dark and there are little rustling sounds all around. I can't see anything and I'm freaking out. I tiptoe carefully through the warehouse. I hear a cat prowling around and then there's a loud crash. I scream. I'm so scared. Then all of a sudden I'm riding across a pond in a horse-drawn sleigh. I'm not sure where we're going, but we're going really fast, almost out of control. It's exhilarating but scary.

Retelling dreams in the present tense sometimes helps clients make dreams more immediate and real and makes the affective components more accessible. This immediacy helps the client reenter the dream and relive the feelings and experience. However, if the client does not want to tell the dream in the first-person present tense, I would not recommend coercing him or her to do so. It is better to let clients set the stage for what they can handle rather than to force them to do what might seem to be too "techniquey" or threatening. The key is to help the client become reimmersed in the dream as much as possible.

Once the client has told the dream, probing about the emotional tone of the dream provides a good starting point for beginning to work with the dream. Asking how the client felt after awakening from the dream can be quite useful, particularly if feelings are unclear from the report. Whether a chase scene left a dreamer feeling terrified or exhilarated makes a difference in the interpretation. For example, a client reported a dream in which he was in the woods with two other people.

They were attacked from behind by werewolves and vampires. He killed one of the vampires and then was knocked unconscious. When he regained consciousness, he saw that his two companions had been killed and laid across each other in an X formation. He knew the legend that if he left them like that, they would become vampires. So he cut their heads off and buried them, making it a sacred ground. I listened to this dream, feeling increasing horror. But when I asked him his feelings when he woke up from the dream, he said that it was not a nightmare but an adventure that he enjoyed. He felt like he was a warrior who was saving the world. He said that he had recently watched the movie *Interview with the Vampire* four times because he enjoyed it so much. Had I followed my assumption that the dream was a nightmare, I would have missed his feelings entirely.

ASSOCIATIONS

Since the time of Freud and Jung, associations have been viewed as a useful intervention to access deep psychic material. Johnson (1986) defined association as "any word, idea, mental picture, feeling, or memory that pops into your mind when you look at the image in the dream" (p. 52). Associating to each image or element of the dream in an affectively laden manner can help the client come to a cognitive and emotional awareness of what the dream means. Associations lead from the image in the dream to the schemata or memory patterns, and thus indicate the issues with which the dreamer is dealing. Through associations, the dreamer can come to understand the schematic connections for each image and see the connections between the event, the dream, and the memories. Central images connecting the dream to past and present issues in waking life typically emerge from this exploratory process.

Each image in the dream comes from the client's individual schemata, so exploration of the images leads directly into the client's thought processes. Associations for each individual will be different because each person has had different experiences and processes information uniquely. In training workshops, we often begin by saying a common word and having everyone in the room say the first thing that comes to their minds. As you would expect, people come up with dramatically different responses to the same word. For example, people might associate "tiger" with a favorite cuddly stuffed toy, a fierce animal, Winnie the Pooh, bedtime stories, tiger in your tank, Calvin and Hobbes, jungle, and so forth. A cuddly stuffed toy typically elicits quite different emotions than does a fierce jungle animal. I cannot emphasize enough that the personal meanings of dream images, rather than universal or standard meanings, are the key to understanding dreams in this model.

Many dreams brought to therapy are bizarre and nonsensical when first presented but make sense when one hears the personal associations to the dream. For example, a dream about a person carrying a mattress on her back across a golf course seemed strange until I heard the dreamer's associations to learning to play golf as a child so that she could have time with her busy father and to always needing to be overprepared wherever she goes.

Importance of Emotions

I would note strongly that associations should not just be sterile cognitions. Emotions are a very important and integral part of the associations. We know that emotional arousal is necessary for change to take place (Frank & Frank, 1991), so it is important to get the client emotionally engaged. Given that emotions are a component of all experience (L. S. Greenberg & Safran, 1987), I postulate that all dreams have emotions attached to them. However, clients are not always in touch with the emotions in dreams. Clients are sometimes blocked emotionally and cannot allow painful feelings to emerge. Typically, once clients can allow the pain to emerge, they can begin to deal with their feelings and thoughts with the support and help of therapists. If clients can begin to experience their emotions, their natural organismic processes can be unlocked and they can become more aware of their potential (see also L. S. Greenberg et al., 1993; Rogers, 1957).

Hence, therapists need to encourage clients to explore their feelings and reactions to dreams thoroughly. By placing oneself back into the dream, a client can get in touch with his or her experience of the affect (Gendlin, 1986; Mahrer, 1990). Too often clients block their feelings because they need to defend themselves against painful emotions. By reexperiencing feelings from dreams in a safe setting, clients can come to accept their feelings. Thus, a major goal of this stage is to enable the client to get back into the dream and to reexperience it in a vivid way to release the associated emotions and cognitions.

Sequential Processing of Major Images

I suggest that therapists progress sequentially through the dream, asking the dreamer to associate to the major images of the dream in the order in which they occurred during the dream. Going through the dream sequentially builds on the natural flow of the dream. Often images that occur later in a dream are derived from the earlier images so that the dream is like a story that unfolds progressively. By going sequentially through their dreams, dreamers have an opportunity to reimmerse themselves in the experience of the dream. They begin to remember the content of the dream and how they felt during the dream. In addition, going sequentially through the dream images seems to simulate the dream formation process in which the person links waking activities to material stored in schemata. Craig and Walsh (1993) present a similar phenomenological approach of reentering the dream and asking for more information about each dream image.

Therapists do not need to cover every image in dreams, especially in long, complicated dreams. Rather, therapists need to pick the images or allow the client to pick the images that seem most central or important to the dreamer. Choosing the important images requires clinical intuition on the therapist's part, but the therapist can check with the client to ensure that the major images have been covered. For example, after going through the images the therapist thinks are important, the therapist can ask the client if he or she would like to explore any additional images.

Direct Associations

I recommend using Jung's (1974) method of association, in which dreamers keep coming back to *specific images* when doing their associations. Coming back to the specific image is in contrast to the more Freudian method of chain association, where one association leads to another, which leads to another (e.g., pumpkin, pie, dinner, family, mother, conflict, anger, etc.). The assumption of the Freudian chain associations is that the person eventually gets to some core conflict. However important this core conflict is for the person, the Jungians point out that the conflict might not have anything to do with the specific dream (see Johnson, 1986). Thus, to determine what the specific image means, therapists should guide the dreamer back to the specific image to generate further associations. For example, a woman who dreamed about a chandelier had many associations to this image, but the associations only began to take on personal meaning when she described the chandelier thoroughly and realized that it was the one that hung in the foyer of her new house. She realized that the chandelier was significant because it represented how uncomfortable she felt in the new, big, elegant house.

Steps of Associations

Describe the Images

The first step in doing associations is to have the client describe each image and the associated feelings more thoroughly. The dream becomes more alive as the client goes through it again and describes each of the images more fully, which is another reason for progressing through the dream sequentially. The dream image for one client was women who were kneeling and praying. When I asked her to describe these women more completely, she suddenly remembered that the women were wearing white dresses. The detail about the white dresses amplified the description of the image. The client said that the women seemed to be nurses. In another example, the dream image was of roller skates. The client described the roller skates as the old metal kind that you wear over your shoes. The idea here is not to have the client give a dry litany of associated words but to get the person involved in talking about what the image means to him or her. Through detailed description of the images, the dreamer begins to relive the dream as it was actually experienced (see also Craig & Walsh, 1993).

Associate to the Images

The next step is for therapists to help clients amplify what the images mean to them through associations. Sometimes therapists need to educate clients briefly about what associations are, give examples, and explain the rationale for doing associations. Associations involve anything the dreamer spontaneously connects to a specific image. Using the example of the dream image of roller skates, examples of possible questions therapists can use to help the client to associate are as follows:

> "What is the first thing that comes to your mind when you think of roller skates?"
> "What do roller skates remind you of?"
> "What might roller skates represent for you?"
> "How are roller skates different from other kinds of skates?"
> "What are roller skates?"
> "How do you feel when you think of roller skates?"
> "What memories do you have of roller skates?"
> "What do you use roller skates for?"
> "Pretend that I am from Mars and have never heard of roller skates. Tell me all about roller skates."

This last prompt comes from Delaney (1991). She suggested that therapists tell clients to pretend that the therapist is from Mars and has never heard of a particular image. The client is asked to explain the image to the therapist. All too often, we assume that we know what an image means to everybody because the word is used commonly. However, when a person has to explain a concept, you begin to realize that this person uses the word differently and has different associations and experiences to it than you do. This method of doing associations encourages the client to explain the image fully without assumptions about what the other person knows.

As an example, in responding to these questions about roller skates, the dreamer indicated that she and her brother had often roller skated as kids. She began talking about the competitiveness that she and her brother had gotten into as kids when roller skating.

As another example, a person dreamed that even though she was late for an appointment, she stopped in the bathroom with her sister to change clothes. I asked her to associate to being late, how she feels when she's late, and if being late reminded her of anything. Then I asked her similar questions about bathrooms, but also asked her if she could remember details about the actual bathroom in the dream. The bathroom was in the Psychology Building, which raised feelings for her about the whole building and about her major and future. Finally, I asked about her sister and about changing clothes, which led to feelings about anger at her sister.

In another example, an elderly nun dreamed that she was watching a mother cat nursing her two kittens. When asked to associate to nursing, her first associations were about nurturance and how much the kittens liked nursing. Upon further reflection, she associated watching the kittens nursing in the dream to feeling that she had not received nurturance as a child from her mother. The associations quickly helped this woman connect with the troubling conflict inside her about her feeling isolated and undernourished. Her metaphor for this feeling may have come from childhood when she watched kittens nursing.

When a person brings up an association, the therapist can reinforce the disclosure and find out more about what the associative material means to him or her. For example, one client presented a dream about being in a chapel in a desert. I asked for associations to chapels, which led to a stream of thoughts about religion. When questioned more about chapels, the client began to talk about his conflicts about being Jewish. When asked about deserts, he associated to the barrenness in his spiritual life and then began to talk about his disagreements with his parents over religion.

If a dreamer is unable to associate to elements in his or her dream, the therapist (or other group members in a group setting) might say what the images would mean if the dreams were his or hers (Ullman & Zimmerman, 1979). In this approach, therapists do not purport to have the "right" association, but rather present possibilities to help clients begin to explore. As with therapist self-disclosure (Hill, Mahalik, & Thompson, 1989), when therapists use their own projections about how they would feel if the dream were theirs, dreamers might feel less threatened and can think about whether the association fits for them. For instance, in a dream of a house with a crumbling foundation, a therapist commented that if the dream were his, he would worry about how stable he felt currently. The client seemed to feel less threatened about this intervention than she would have if the therapist had said that the dream revealed that the client was unstable. In a group therapy setting, having everyone associate to the different elements "as if it were my dream" can lead to valuable insights for both the dreamer and the other group members. This projection exercise can also help normalize feelings and create group cohesion. (See Chapter 11 for an example of projection in a dream group.) It is crucial to remember, however, that associations given by another person may not have meaning for the dreamer. Hence, others should always own that the associations are theirs and may or may not fit for the dreamer.

Therapists should not assume that they know what images mean for clients. Even if he or she is accurate about what an image means based on his or her knowledge of a client, the therapist has not allowed the client the opportunity to explore the image and come to his or her own understanding and ownership. Furthermore, if the interpretation of an image is taken from a dream dictionary (e.g., all snakes are phallic objects), it may not apply for a particular client and can bring personal exploration to a halt. Dreamers often then look to their therapists for explanations of the meaning of images rather than looking inwards for their own explanations.

Evoking Emotional Arousal

Clients will often become very involved in reexperiencing the dream simply by going back through the dream sequentially and associating to the images in the dream. However, the therapist may need to prod the client to get into the feelings more completely. The following two techniques are often useful for evoking greater emotional arousal.

Experience the Feeling

If a person mentions a strong feeling in a dream but is not currently experiencing that feeling, we might ask him or her to focus on it and experience it more fully (Gendlin, 1986; Mahrer, 1990). Experiencing the feelings in dreams can help dreamers come to accept feelings as parts of themselves. In addition, once a person can allow the feeling to occur fully, it typically then flows into a new feeling. It is only when the feeling is blocked from occurrence that it does not evolve. For example, one person's dream revealed sadness over a bird's death. I asked him to try to stay with the sadness more and tell us about the feelings. It was difficult for him to get into the sadness, but as he did he became aware of his continuing and unresolved grief over his mother's death. By staying with the grief, he was able to experience other feelings toward his mother, including anger and caring.

Be the Image

Another method to help a person get more into feelings is to have him or her "be" the part or image in the dream. For example, a person who dreamed of a car was asked to be the car. He said, "I'm sporty, fast, bright red, and new. Everyone notices me but underneath there's a leak. I can't find out what is wrong, but I'm afraid that I will blow up." Being the image can help the dreamer reexperience the dream more vividly and come to accept the feelings as part of him- or herself.

LINKS TO WAKING LIFE

A fair amount of evidence now exists that dreams reflect waking life (see review in Chapter 2). Thus, when something happens during the day that arouses us in some way, particularly negatively, we tend to dream about the event(s) at night in metaphorical form. By identifying the triggering event(s) that led to the dream, therapists can begin to help clients understand their feelings and reactions to the event(s). By using associations, clients can also be helped to understand how their reactions to present events are related to memories of similar events in the past. Thus, once therapists have a sense of what a dream image means to the client, they need to be attentive to discovering the connections or links to waking life.

Clients often spontaneously make links to waking life while they are doing the associations. If they do not spontaneously make the links, therapists can systematically go back through the images and ask clients for the links after they have completed the associations. Referring to the notes that he or she has taken of the major images, the therapist can ask about whether the image and related associations remind the client of anything that has been happening recently in his or her waking life. For example, one part of a dream involved a truck careening wildly out of control down the highway. The dreamer's associations to the image of the truck were of being out of control, anxiety, exhilaration, and panic. I asked if there was anything in the dreamer's life that felt like it was careening wildly out of control and making her anxious but excited. The client responded that her moods felt like that lately. By exploring this connection further, we were able to see how the dream reflected what was going on in her life at the time. In another example, a dreamer's association to the image of oils sitting on a dusty shelf in a Mexican general store was of healing spirits tucked away in an out-of-the-way spot. Her connection of these associations to her waking life was that she had life-giving potentials that she had been hiding away and that she needed to dust them off and use them.

Therapists might also want to find out more about the client's memories during this section of the interpretation process. For example, if a client mentions her father in the associations, the therapist might want to pursue this topic further and find out what kind of relationship the client had with her father. Similarly, an event in the dream that is typically related to a key developmental point in the client's life might suggest probing the events of that period. For example, a therapist trainee was doubtful that we would be able to do much with a fragment of a dream she had about her teeth falling out. After associating to the image of teeth and teeth falling out, we asked the dreamer what was happening in her life around the time when her teeth fell out. She responded that her teeth fell out in early childhood. She then began to talk about her early childhood and revealed a number of very salient unresolved issues that still troubled her from that time period. We spent over an hour processing this small fragment of a dream because of the richness of her associations and the links to past events.

Once the therapist helps the client make the link of the dream element to waking life and explores that issue, he or she generally will want to bring the process back to the dream. Typically, a clinical decision is involved in whether to stick with the movement that one is making on a particular issue or whether to return to the dream. Obviously, if the issue is important, the therapist will want to continue where there is therapeutic movement. However, it is important to come back to trying to understand the totality of the dream. Analyzing the whole dream often leads to a different understanding than just looking at some elements in isolation.

WORKING WITH CONFLICTS IN DREAMS

Often a dreamer either has difficulty reexperiencing the emotions in the dream or has strong conflicts that get aroused by the dream. Rather than proceeding to the Insight Stage, working with these conflicts directly can be useful in bringing about a greater exploration of feelings and thoughts.

Because dreams often reveal underlying conflicts, working with this conflictual material in therapy can provide the opportunity for self-exploration, which can lead to greater self-understanding. During the Exploration Stage, therapists can look for markers that indicate the presence of an unresolved conflict (L. S. Greenberg et al., 1993), such as resistance to exploring a particular image, a split between two different feelings, or unresolved grief. Working with the conflict directly and experientially can facilitate an awareness of all the components of the conflict and can also facilitate resolution.

Therapists might have clients dialogue with or enact the different parts in the dream, as suggested by Gestalt (e.g., Yontef & Simkin, 1989) and Jungian theorists (e.g., Johnson, 1986). Working with the conflicts can be particularly useful as a way of getting clients more in touch with their feelings. For example, one student in a training workshop had a dream that she was observing her dead body being carried down the stairs. This conflict split provided an excellent opportunity to have her observing side dialogue with her dead body, thus having her clarify the feelings and get more in touch with the two sides of herself.

One client's dream reflected a conflict with his father over religion; his father wanted him to be a traditional Jew, whereas he was more interested in exploring alternative religions. In addition, his father was authoritarian and wanted his son to do everything his way. I asked the client to pretend that his father was in the empty chair and talk to him. As he spoke to his father in the empty chair and then reversed roles and spoke as his father, the conflict between the father's dominance and the son's desire to be his own person became clearer. Through role playing and experiencing the affect of both sides of the conflict and making sure that each side listened to the other side, some understanding and resolution was possible (see also L. S. Greenberg & Dompierre, 1981; L. S. Greenberg & Higgins, 1980). My client was able to speak up to his "father" during the role play and tell him that he needed to make his own decisions. His "father" was able to listen and tolerate the client's speaking up, which gave the client some hope that in fact his real father would listen if he were able to tell him how he felt.

In another example, a client related a dream about a rosebush. I asked her to be the rosebush. She said,

I'm growing on both sides of the fence. One side is in my parents' yard. The other side is in the neighbor's yard. I feel split between the two sides. On my parents' side, I feel trapped but safe. On the neighbor's side, I feel beautiful but scared.

Thus, she described a split or a conflict in her feelings. After going through the associations and links to waking life, I asked her to be the bush on the neighbor's side and tell the bush on her parents' side how she felt. She talked about wanting to feel attractive but not wanting to go too far away. Then she became the rose on the parents' side and talked about wanting to be there to take care of her parents but not feel so much like a child. She acted out both sides until she reached a compromise, which was that she wanted to stay on the fence but to interweave the two sides. Instead of an ugly chain link fence showing, she wanted to beautify both yards while staying grounded in who she was.

Alternatively, therapists might ask dreamers to paint, sing, or dance to express more fully some part of the dream that they are having trouble understanding or that is of particular salience to them. Of course, therapists need to be trained in using such techniques and clients need to be open to using them. For example, an artistic client in brief therapy painted the images from her recurrent dream after she and the therapist had spent several sessions working with the dream. Interestingly, the painting looked very different from her original dream because the images had transformed as she worked on the dream. Bringing the painting in to the final session was a powerful way of discussing the changes the client had made through examining the recurrent dream.

For therapists and clients who are comfortable using them, these nonverbal activities enable dreamers to go beyond the verbal responses typically used as the sole medium in counseling and therapy. In a sense, such nonverbal activities are close to a replication of the dream experience. Once clients have done the activity, therapists can ask them to articulate what they have learned, enabling clients to put nonverbal experiences into words and integrate these different modes of cognitive processing.

We should note that therapists might not always work with conflicts in doing dream interpretation. In my experience, the need to work intensively with conflicts is less universal than the need to work with the feelings and associations. It is useful, however, for therapists to be prepared to help clients work with conflicts to get more out of the Exploration Stage.

THERAPIST TECHNIQUES THAT FACILITATE EXPLORATION

In this method, therapists try to facilitate clients in coming to their own understanding of the meaning of the dream. Thus, therapists are directive in that they follow a definite structure of processing the images, but they are not directive in the sense of telling clients what the dream means or what to do about the dream. Therapists are nondirective in the sense that they have no particular associations to which they are trying to lead the client. Thus, in this stage therapists try to stay within the client's framework to allow clients to explore their schemata. Perhaps the best description is that therapists are directive of the process but not of the outcome.

As an example, a student who I was training to use the model was working very hard to present various associations and feelings to the client. The client was sitting passively, not very involved in the process and feeling that the therapist did not quite understand her. I suggested to the therapist that she step back and allow the client to do the associating. She could facilitate the client getting into the associations by using fairly minimal, open-ended questions and reflections. When she tried this approach, the client immediately got involved and began exploring the dream images.

There are a number of helpful basic skills that therapists can use to facilitate client exploration. I discuss these briefly to show that dream interpretation is not magical but consists of basic skills that all therapists should have in their repertoire. These skills are covered in greater depth in other texts (e.g., Benjamin, 1981; Egan, 1986; L. S. Greenberg et al., 1993; Ivey, 1995) and are based on my previous research on therapist techniques (see review in Hill, 1992).

Open-Ended Questions

Open-ended questions are the primary tool that therapists will use to elicit associations. Therapists have to suspend their own projections and thoughts about the images and lead clients through a series of open-ended questions to help them connect the image with their personal associations. Examples include the following:

"What is an elevator?"
"I wonder how you feel when you imagine yourself in a white BMW convertible?"
"What is your experience of your mother when she walks like that?"

Therapists do not have a particular answer in mind when asking these open-ended questions but rather are encouraging clients to explore their own thoughts. Open-ended questions require dreamers to explore what they are thinking and feeling with minimal cues from the therapist about what they "should" be saying, so therapists should be aware that this type of question can be threatening for some clients who try too hard to please their therapists (see Hill, 1989, 1992; Hill et al., 1988). It is crucial that questions be asked in a gentle, respectful manner rather than being done rapidly with no concern for the client.

Reflection of Feelings

Once a client has associated to an image, the therapist can reflect the feelings associated with the image so that the client becomes or stays immersed in the experience of the dream. Once again, we are not so concerned with having the client generate numerous associations to a particular image as we are with having the client associate to what the image and the associated feelings were like in the particular dream. Enabling the dreamer to reexperience the affect helps him or her begin to accept and understand the feelings. Furthermore, it allows all the affective/cognitive components of the schemata to be activated so that the dreamer can become more aware of his or her reactions and memories that are stimulated by the image. Examples include the following:

"You sound upset right now like you might want to cry when you picture the dead flowers."

"Seeing your brother get married must have been exciting for you."

"I wonder if you felt relieved because you were able to avoid drinking when you saw that whole wall of booze in your dream."

Reflection of feelings is an ideal therapist technique for helping dreamers get into the emotional aspect of images. Reflection of feelings serves several functions beyond getting the dreamer to reexperience the dream (see also Egan, 1986; L. S. Greenberg et al., 1993; Hill, 1989, 1992; Hill et al., 1988; Vossen, 1990). Reflections indicate to the client that the therapist is actively attempting to understand the client's experience. Rather than making clients do all the work, therapists are collaboratively involved in trying to pinpoint client feelings. If therapists present the reflections tentatively (e.g., "I wonder whether you feel anxious about the stairs melting away"), clients are encouraged to try on the feeling to see if it fits with their inner experience. Reflections also force therapists to try to communicate their understanding of the client's feelings. Having to reflect the feelings challenges therapists to see whether they actually do understand what clients are expressing and provides the opportunity for them to get feedback about misunderstandings. For clients, hearing a reflection of what they have been saying can force them to rethink and describe more precisely what they really feel. Of course it is important that the therapist tries to imagine how the client must feel and deliver the reflection in a deeply empathic manner. Reflections that are delivered in a standardized, robotic manner are clearly not helpful.

Attending Behaviors

Minimal encouragers ("Mm hmm," "I see," "Go ahead") and inviting nonverbal behaviors (head nods, appropriate eye contact) are crucial during all phases of the treatment, but especially during the Exploration Stage. These behaviors typically communicate to the client that the therapist is engaged; they also help to keep the client involved in the demanding task of exploring associations and emotional reactions.

Rarely Used Interventions

During the Exploration Stage, therapists would rarely, if ever, use interpretations or confrontations. Furthermore, therapists would seldom give information or advice about what to do outside the session. Interpretations, confrontations, information, and direct guidance could all deflect from the primary goal of facilitating client involvement in the exploration process.

AMOUNT OF TIME NEEDED
FOR EXPLORATION STAGE

The length and complexity of the dream, as well as the dreamer's ability to elaborate on the images, dictates how long therapists will need to spend in the Exploration Stage. A simple dream might take just a few minutes for the client to explore, especially if the client is not elaborative and open to exploring the metaphorical parts of the dream. If, on the other hand, the dream is long and complicated, 2 to 3 hours might be needed to explore it thoroughly. Therapists need to spend as long as necessary to gain an understanding of what the images mean to the individual dreamer.

EXTENDED EXAMPLE:
QUEEN FOR A DREAM

The following is an example of a therapist and client going through the Exploration Stage. The client was a 44-year-old woman whose marriage had been annulled. She had a high school education and did child care in her home. She came to therapy because she had pain and depression stemming from an accident, nervousness with the children she was responsible for in her child-care job, and anger at her ex-husband. She was currently on medication (Prozac and occasionally Xanax). The therapist was a 40-year-old, master's-level, licensed male counselor who had a Jungian orientation and 10 years of clinical experience. This session was the 9th of 12 sessions of a successful case of brief individual therapy conducted for the Diemer, Lobell, Vivino, and Hill (1996) study (see Chapter 12 for more details about this study). The client and therapist both read the transcript of this session and gave consent for it to be used in this book.

The transcript has been edited to make it shorter and easier to read, but the meaning of the dialogue has not been altered. C stands for client and T stands for therapist in the transcript. Figure 5.1 shows the major images and associations that were generated in the Exploration Stage.

The Dream

I'm walking down a road, and I come upon the most beautiful place I've ever seen. It's truly majestic. It's a panorama of green all around. There are white castles off in the distance. I am struck by how beautiful this scene is. I continue to walk down this road and come across a memorial of sorts. There are three or four rows of soldiers, almost like from the Nutcracker Suite. *I'm wondering who's being honored and then realize it's the Air Force.*

T: Tell me a little more about the place.

C: I just remember a lot of green trees, green grass, it's just green everywhere. Then, not the full view of the castle, more or less like the tops, the turrets. I just knew they were castles by that.

T: Let's start with the green. When you think of green, what comes to mind?

C: Money (*laugh*), lots of it, too. There was lots of green in my dream.

T: Okay, lots of money. What else?

C: Well, vegetation, vegetables, healthy.

T: What else? Think a little bit further than that. What else comes up besides money, healthy, and vegetation?

C: Well, I've always heard it was a calming color, too. That's why doctors' offices are painted green.

T: Calming color. Was it calming to you in the dream?

C: Yeah, very calming. It was just like I was thinking, "Wow, this so beautiful." I was peaceful.

Images	Associations
Green	Money, vegetation, vegetables, healthy, calming color, doctor's office
Lush green vegetation	Gardens down south, plenty of food to eat
Beautiful places	Desire to travel, castles in England
Soldiers	3–4 rows, marching in place, nutcrackers, protection, security
Dress uniforms	Authority, higher position, control over others, dated a policeman
Castles	I belong in a castle, splendor, living royally, beautiful, big, magnificent, queen of the castle, people do stuff for you, position of authority
Air Force	Up higher, spirituality, protection
Memorials	To honor, D.C. memorials, Dad's grave, to pay tribute to someone great after they're dead, captured in time

FIGURE 5.1. A grid for recording images and associations with examples taken from the excerpted session.

T: What about the lush green vegetation? What is that?

C: When I lived down south as a little girl, we always had gardens growing, and there was always a lot of green, so I remember that. We just went down there not too long ago. There is green everywhere.

T: Was the landscape in your dream similar to the area down South?

C: No, this was more flat.

T: So you could see a long-off distance?

C: Yeah, it was way off in the distance that I could see these castles. I don't know even if it was a road, but I was walking along a path or something and just came upon this scene.

T: Tell me more about the vegetation. I want you to associate. What does lush vegetation bring to mind?

C: Plenty of food to eat.

T: Okay, plenty to eat. (*pause*) You're walking down the path and going through all this lush greenery. What were you feeling?

C: I just remember feeling very calm and peaceful and thinking "Wow, this is just the most beautiful place I've ever seen." I wouldn't be surprised if somebody had told me the next morning that I said that out loud in the middle of the night. It was that vivid, like I was just really there.

T: What's your association to beautiful places?

C: (*sigh*) I've never seen anything like it. It brings to mind some place I'd like to go that I've never been, especially with the castle. I've seen some beautiful scenery in the U.S., but nothing like what was in my dream.

T: Do you have a sense of where it was?

C: From the castles, maybe England. I'm walking just a little past what is like the Air Force. They were like real men, only they were dressed up in their dress clothes. I'm thinking, "Wow, this is some kind of memorial, what could this be?" Then something told me it's the Air Force. It's like, "Oh man, what does that mean?"

T: Tell me a little bit more about the soldiers. Can you describe them?

C: I can't describe any specifically. I just know there were three or four rows of them, and they were marching in place.

T: Nutcracker uniforms?

C: That's what it reminded me of. That's what I thought of the next morning when I was thinking of that.

T: What color were they?

C: I remember a lot of blues.

T: When you think of soldiers, what comes to mind?

C: Protection, security. They're going to protect you from someone who is coming to try to hurt you. Just being secure knowing that they're watching out for you. What else do I think of it as? They wear dress uniforms, too. It would almost be majestic because they do wear the uniforms and they weren't in fatigues or anything like that.

T: Tell me about dress uniforms.

C: Someone who has authority, one of a higher position, someone who has control over others.

T: Security, protection, control over others.

C: Yeah, once I dated a policeman, and I felt very secure when I was with him. (laugh) It was like if you get in trouble, you call the police, right, and he's right here, so I can't possibly be scared. He even had a gun there on the table, which I'd never touch. Actually he wasn't in a uniform either. He was a plainclothes, but I still thought of it that way.

T: But here you had a whole army of soldiers to protect you.

C: Right.

T: What about the castles? What comes to mind when you think of castles?

C: Well, I've just always said because I'm a Leo, I feel like I belong in a castle. (laugh) That's where I should be, in a castle, like splendor and . . .

T: Splendor. What else?

C: This sounds bad, but having other people do all your stuff for you, (laugh) but not even that so much as just living royally.

T: Royally.

C: Yeah, it's all very nice. Like in my house I'm always saying, "God, I wish I could fix that so it didn't look like that." But if I were royal, I wouldn't have to do that.

T: In a castle, everything is nice.

C: Right.

T: Anything else about castles?

C: I suppose there is the position of authority again too, but mostly just the fact that it's beautiful and really big and magnificent. I should be in a big room with Queen Victoria's bed or something. Instead, I'm sleeping in a bed with no headboard. I feel like I deserve better.

T: So in your dream there's a lot of imagery. There's a lot of association with beauty, with plushness, with luxury. It's safe. It's calm. It's protected.

C: It's just what I would like, all of that. Yeah, exactly.

T: What about the Air Force? What does that bring to mind?

C: At first, I'm thinking that's so crazy, but then afterwards, I realized I had this dream last week after we talked about how I would like to meet some people who are into spirituality and not so down to earth, so I thought that maybe the fact that they were the Air Force, they're up higher.

T: Okay.

C: Plus last week we had talked about how I'm the master of my fate, I'm the captain of my soul. It's like if I lived in a castle, I would be the master.

T: Queen of the castle.

C: Right. When I say other people under me, I don't necessarily mean it to be mean to them or anything, but just other people who are there to serve you (*laugh*) and make your life really nice.

T: That's real appealing.

C: Right (*laugh*), yes.

T: You're protected, served, and surrounded by everything that's beautiful, the most beautiful place you've ever been.

C: I always have felt like I should be a queen or at least a princess.

T: And here it was.

C: Right.

T: Anything else about the Air Force, besides it being spiritual, higher, and a higher plane?

C: In the Air Force their uniforms are blue and white, the way I was thinking of them, and just the fact that they're up high, so that they're protecting you from enemies who are really far away.

T: Sort of a cosmic protection on a higher plane?

C: Yeah (*laugh*), no pun intended, right?

T: The pun was definitely intended. I see one more image that we need to talk about. You said there was a memorial to the Air Force.

C: Right.

T: What are your associations to memorials?

C: Honor, to honor them, to pay tribute, almost the same thing, to pay homage to. It was almost like I was in D.C. looking at some of the memorials, although this was real men. But it's just like I realized this is a memorial, who is it for, just to honor or an organization, the whole organization?

T: What else about memorials?

C: I don't know. Maybe when I went down to my Dad's grave, I felt like his grave should have looked nicer. It was a memorial to him. Actually on top of his grave was all green too, and we had to pull it all up and put down some other stuff and some flowers around. It was like a memorial to him.

T: It's not just *like* a memorial, it is a memorial.

C: Right. I felt like it should have looked nicer. It makes me feel a little sad that we don't make it look nice all the time, but it's so far away. We decided that we're going to go back again next year and do it even nicer. This time I took stuff with me, but I didn't have enough of some of the things that I needed to make it look really nice.

T: Anything else about a memorial that comes to mind? If I were from Mars and never heard of a memorial, what would you tell me a memorial is?

C: (*sigh*) Mostly the things that I just said, that it's to pay tribute to someone who has done something great, something worth remembering, and it's there for all the world to see, that these people were great, and to honor them long after they die.

T: Memorial comes from the same root as memory. It has to do with memory and remembering.

C: Right. I always say I don't want my picture taken because I don't want to be memorialized. I don't want the picture 20 years from now.

T: So the image is something that's captured in time and held still.

C: Right. So I try to skip by these few years that I've looked so horrible. Those were my years "in the black." As the poem says, "Out of the night that covers me, black as the pit from pole to pole." That's how I felt, how I had felt in the past, but I feel like I'm coming out of that.

T: Is that a part of your life that you'd like to forget about, not memorialize?

C: I don't want to forget about it actually because I feel like I've done something good by overcoming it all, and because I've always heard that to help other people you need to have gone through it yourself. I feel like 20 or 30 years from now I can help other people by knowing what it's like.

T: So you wouldn't mind memorializing that part of your life?

C: Right, in fact I've just been thinking maybe I should start taking some astrologic notes about this Pluto transit that I'm going through. It's perfect because it shows exactly what the textbook would show you. It's happened the way the textbook would tell you, yet when you read it and you're not going through it, it's hard to understand. So I'm going to try to make some notes of my own to go along with the book. Not only that, but I started thinking about other things in astrology of keeping notes on too, just to memorialize it so that 20 years from now I'll have that and not try to just keep it all in my head.

T: It's interesting that you've talked several times about Pluto transit.

Both of your dreams had some of the events that you've talked about in your life. There's been a lot of themes having to do with death or graves or cemeteries. Death seems to be a very important theme. It's interesting that even in this dream, which is the most beautiful place you've ever seen, it's all beauty and plushness, yet there's still a place for a memorial because I think that's important to you. No matter how much your life improves, how good things get, you still need a place that's set aside for death and all the aspects of what death means.

C: Yeah, because actually Pluto is like a death of an old self and a rebirth of a new self.

T: If you look at the word, the original Latin word "Pluto" means wealth.

C: I didn't know that.

T: The underworld is where all the food and crops grow. They come from under the ground. So it's the underworld that is the source of the plushness, the lush greenery, and all that.

C: I didn't know that. I just knew through astrology that Pluto can be rising out of the ashes, the Phoenix bird rising out of it's own ashes into the light, or into the heights.

T: How does that relate to you and this dream?

C: I do feel like in the last couple months I've improved a lot, and maybe this is showing me what is to come, this beautiful place. Maybe it's just the whole earth, maybe it's just going to be my view of things around me, that this is really a beautiful place. It's probably the first time I ever really thought of it that way.

T: Let's work with the feelings that come with the different imagery there. You're in the most beautiful place you've ever seen, lush greenery, castles.

C: I'm feeling really calm and peaceful. In the last 10 years mostly what I've wanted is to feel calm and peaceful. I've said it so many times, "I would just like to have peace of mind and to be calm." I have calmed myself down over the last couple months since I've been coming here and since I've been going to acupuncture. I've felt much calmer than I had in the past.

T: Put yourself back in the place where you were in the dream, in the greenery and the road with all the lushness, and just be there for a minute. What's that like?

C: It's serene. Peaceful is the best word to describe it.

T: Can you describe the landscape in any more detail?

C: Just remember a lot of green, all the grass was really green, and trees, but not a mountain, just a lot of trees, and then the white castles, just the tops of them all.

T: If you were one of those trees, what might you say to yourself?

C: Come on over and sit in the shade. Sit down awhile and rest, would you?

T: Anything else the tree might want to say? Do you have a message for her?

C: Just welcome. It's about time you got here. (*pause*) Where is your crown?

T: Okay, the other one. As yourself, what do you say back to the trees?

C: It's really nice to be here. It's so quiet and peaceful. I would like to stay here for hours. I want to be peaceful forever.

T: Okay, now you're the tree again. Would you say anything else?

C: You're here now, so don't go back, stay here. Stay with us, we'll protect you, we'll love you, or, we'll protect you, you'll be happy here.

T: Okay, as you one more time, respond to the tree.

C: You've talked me into it. I'm never leaving. I could be happy here. I love the trees. I love all the green. I love the feeling I have when I'm here. I like feeling this way.

T: How are you feeling?

C: Calm and peaceful and serene and just like nothing could ever happen that could make me feel bad if I stay here, just going to always feel good.

T: Do you want to stay?

C: I would like to, yeah. I used to say I would like to go up to the mountains into a cabin where nobody knew who I was and just live there because then I felt like I could be calm and by myself.

T: It's interesting in the dream you didn't stay there, you kept walking down the path away from the castle. What drew you to leave this calm, serene tree to go to the memorial?

C: It's like I have a place to go that I wasn't aware of. There's someplace I'm supposed to go, walking down this road, and this is what I see. Even though I love this place, it's like I still have to go. When I got to the memorial I was trying to interpret what this means, this thing here, like, "I know this is a memorial, but what is it for?" Then I don't know if I see a sign that says Air Force or just intuitively know that this is to memorialize the Air Force.

T: What did the memorial look like? Was there a structure there?

C: No, basically there were just these rows of soldiers.

T: So they were the memorial?

C: Right, there was no structure at all. I don't know why I'm calling it a memorial. That's what I was calling it in my dream.

T: That's what it felt like to you.

C: Right.

T: Is there something you'd like to ask the memorial, you'd like to ask one of the soldiers? Anything else you want to know?

C: Why are you in my dream? Why am I dreaming about the Air Force?

T: Now let yourself be that memorial. Take a minute to imagine yourself as the memorial. Answer your question.

C: We're just here to let you know we'll always protect you. We will just always be here with you to protect you and make sure that nothing ever happens to you. Even if you don't know who we are, we're still going to protect you.

T: Did that answer your question?

C: Yeah, sort of. What I have felt before at times when I've been in trouble, just I know I can always count on myself. That when I can count on no one else, I can always count on me. So maybe the forces are in me, but I just forgot that for awhile.

T: You have some rows of soldiers inside of you?

C: Yeah, the poem made me realize that. Have you ever heard the whole poem?

T: Yeah.

C: I feel like it was written by me or for me.

T: Well, a captain has to have soldiers, right?

C: Right. After I thought about it awhile, it's like the master's for the castle, and the captain's for the soldiers. So I'm the captain of my soul, and my soldiers are there to help me. Actually one part of the line is, "I thank whatever gods may be for my unconquerable soul." I feel like with all that I've been through in the last 10 years, some other people might have given in to it. There are many, many times when I wanted to or did maybe by just crying and feeling sad and alone and all that, but I basically never gave up. There was like an underlying feeling of hope there somewhere.

T: Is there anything else you want to say to the memorial?

C: I'm glad you're here with me. I'll be a good captain. I'll never steer you wrong.

T: Is there anything you'd like to ask the Air Force?

C: I don't know if there's anything I want to ask, but my favorite brother was in the Air Force. All my other brothers were in the Army.

T: He's not in the Air Force any more?

C: No, but I remember when he was in the Air Force. I remember when I was a little girl him paying a lot of attention to me.

T: Did you ever see him in his uniform?

C: My mother used to have pictures of all of them in uniforms.

T: What does that mean to you that your brother was in the Air Force?

C: All of my brothers did their duty. I don't know why my one brother chose the Air Force. I think it's because he wanted to go overseas. He probably wanted to get as far away from that little town we were from as possible. I guess I would like to go all over to all those places.

T: Just do the traveling around the world. Have you done any traveling around the world?

C: I went to Jamaica. (*laugh*) That's about as far as I've gotten. But I'd like to go like really far away to Spain, and France, and Australia, and other places. There's probably some really beautiful places that I haven't seen yet that I would like to see, far away from where I came from.

T: You didn't make it to the castle, right?

C: No, there wasn't even a feeling of wanting to go to the castle.

T: What were you most drawn to?

C: Just the serenity of it all, just so calm and peaceful, just so, "Wow, this is great, it's so beautiful." The next morning the word that came to my mind was majestic, just this big wide shot, like CinemaScope almost.

T: What's majestic about you? Tell me about your majesty.

C: My soul, maybe not my outside appearance, but my soul is majestic.

T: Can you describe it for me? What's majestic about it?

C: Just it's on a higher plane. (*laugh*) It's (*pause*) away from the earth. It's not earth like this. My soul is like cosmopolitan or universal, wants to know all, and wants to learn what I need to learn to become better as far as lessons and learning.

T: Can you tell me that again with a majestic voice?

C: Let's see. I am a higher soul. I'm not talking like a queen, am I? I AM A HIGHER SOUL. I WANT TO DO GOOD. I WANT TO DO GOOD FOR ALL MY SUBJECTS. I WANT TO LEARN FROM THEM AND TEACH THEM AND BE A BETTER PERSON.

T: Who are your subjects?

C: All those who know me, who learn from me, who come in contact with me, who I try to help by sharing what I do, what I have learned, what I know, or what I've learned. But I don't want to be the queen so that I can rule everyone and make them do exactly what I want them to do. It's just I want to make them better people.

T: Serve the realm. That's really the goal of the true queen—to serve the realm. Another term is to shepherd the realm, sometimes they call it that.

C: Right, that's what I would like. But I also get to live a very good life, too, in a beautiful castle with guards all around to protect me.

T: What would that mean in your life, to live in a castle with lush greenery and guards to protect you?

C: Just means doing better than I'm doing right now financially—a beautiful house, nice furniture. I want more than just what you need to get by with.

Commentary

This example is a good illustration of the Exploration Stage because the therapist used lots of different interventions to explore the dream, including retelling the dream, associations, intensifying the affect, linking the images to waking life, and working with conflicts in the dream. This therapist did an especially good job of working with the client's affect. The therapist was generally very facilitative of encouraging the client come to her own associations. In a couple of instances, however, he cut off the client's exploration by telling her what particular dream images meant, for example, telling her that memorial comes from the root word of memory and so has to do with memory and remembering and indicating that, in the original Latin, Pluto means wealth. But the therapist did a good job of bringing the focus back and asking the client how these meanings fit for her dream.

The relationship between the therapist and client seemed strong. The therapist was very supportive, and the alliance seemed collaborative. He was accepting, in that he did not argue with the client's beliefs in spiritualism, astrology, and acupuncture. Instead, he allowed the client to explore how these beliefs were related to her dream.

In the remainder of the session (not excerpted in this book), the therapist asked the client to talk about what the different parts of the dream meant. The client was able to identify how she was changing and feeling more in charge of her life, more like the master of the ship or the queen of the castle. The therapist helped the client integrate what she learned from the dream by asking her to think about how she wanted to be different. The therapist ended by suggesting that she read about (or watch a movie about) some queen to give her someone with whom to identify. Interpreting this dream helped the client realize that she had more resources than she thought she had and that she could be in charge of her life.

When I contacted her over 2 years after the termination of therapy to obtain permission to use portions of the transcript in this book, the client indicated that she still thought about the work in therapy on this specific dream. She had been wanting to take a vacation to the Caribbean, but felt she could not afford it. She had been thinking about her need for peace and serenity. Reading the transcript gave her the impetus to decide to take the vacation.

SUMMARY

In summary, Exploration is the most important stage in this model because it sets the foundation for the stages to follow. Because dreams connect waking events and past memories, they are unique to each person and hence can only be understood by processing them thoroughly with the person. Through associations that are done with emotional arousal, the dreamer is able to go back and activate the relevant schemata so that they can be restructured. The therapist needs to have a firm grounding in what each image means to the client to arrive at a helpful interpretation of the dream. Throughout the exploration process, the therapist is teaching the client valuable skills for carefully exploring his or her feelings, thoughts, and reactions to each piece of the dream. The Exploration Stage proceeds through having the client retell the dream, asking sequentially for associations to the dream images, evoking emotional arousal, linking the images to waking life, and perhaps working with conflicts.

CHAPTER SIX

Insight Stage

O NCE THE DREAM has been explored thoroughly, therapists can move to the Insight Stage. In this stage, the therapist tries to help the client "put it all together" and figure out what the dream means. Therapists can help clients achieve greater self-understanding by integrating what clients have learned through self-exploration into an interpretation of the dream. Understanding dreams is important because of the potential to yield greater self-awareness and problem resolution. Integrating the understanding of the parts of the dream from the Exploration Stage brings the dreamer to a new level of awareness and insight. Table 6.1 shows the goals of this stage, the tasks to be accomplished, the most frequently used and rarely used therapist techniques, and the desired therapist manner.

THEORY ABOUT INSIGHT

Most psychodynamic theorists believe that insight is an important mechanism of change in the therapy process. Action without insight would be sterile because the client would not have any understanding of his or her behavior. The person would be more like an automaton rather than a creature striving to make sense out of his or her world.

What Is Insight?

Elliott et al. (1994) described four aspects of insight: metaphorical vision (seeing oneself in a new light), connection (perceptions of patterns or links often involving reasons, causes, categorizations, or parallels), suddenness (a feeling of surprise or "Aha"), and newness (a sense of discovery). Clients often experience these four aspects with a feeling that the interpretation "clicks," "feels right," and helps them understand something they did not understand before. Thus, insight involves coming to some new understanding about oneself.

Singer (1965) noted that insight needs to be both intellectual and experiential to have an impact. If insight is just intellectual, it has a barren quality and often leads to clients feeling stuck in an analytic understanding that leads nowhere. On the other hand, if insight has an emotional component, the client is more likely to feel it at a greater depth and with more of a sense of personal involvement.

Through exploration of thoughts and feelings in collaboration with a therapist, clients often arrive naturally at insight into their dreams. Insight usually involves a greater understanding of the dream and thus helps to integrate sleeping and waking, past and present, conscious and unconscious material. Dreams often reveal feelings or thoughts that

---

TABLE 6.1. Outline for the Insight Stage

I. Goals

    A. Use data from Exploration Stage to facilitate understanding.
    B. Try to determine the meaning of the dream for the client.
    C. Restructure client's schemata to accommodate new data.
    D. Use own experience to foster client awareness.
    E. Maintain the therapeutic alliance.

II. Tasks

    A. Introduce the Insight Stage.
        1. Ask about the meaning of the dream.
        2. Restate the dream using the associations (optional).
    B. Collaborate with client to understand dream using one or more of the four possible levels of interpretation:
        1. Dream experience
        2. Relation to current waking events
        3. Relation to past memories
        4. Parts of self
    C. Have client summarize the meaning of the dream.

III. Therapist techniques

    A. Frequently used techniques: Open-ended question, reflection of feelings, minimal encourager
    B. Less frequently used but important techniques: Interpretation, confrontation
    C. Rarely used techniques: Information, direct guidance

IV. Therapist manner

    A. Collaborative
    B. Facilitative

---

clients were not aware of and now must try to fit into their perceptions of themselves. An interpretation can give a dreamer a new understanding of him- or herself both through assimilating new learning into existing schemata and by adapting existing schemata to accommodate the new material (see Field, Barkham, Shapiro, & Stiles, 1994; Stiles, Barkham, Shapiro, & Firth-Cozens, 1992; Stiles et al., 1990; Stiles, Meshot, Anderson, & Sloan, 1992). Additionally, the changes in schemata allow the person to behave differently in the world.

Restructuring Schemata through Insight

One of the major changes that is often accomplished by insight is a change in the dreamer's schemata. Once the dreamer brings the schemata into full awareness through the associations and the emotional arousal, he or she begins to rethink assumptions and thought patterns. The possibility of change seems to be greatest when a schema is fully activated. The dreamer has some motivation at that time to reexamine what he or she has expected or believes. For example, a person may have had a firm belief that she received inadequate parenting, which left her unable to cope with life. Through examination of the evocative associations to images in a dream about cuddling a newborn child, a dreamer may come to a powerful realization that she is able to give nurturance to others and that in fact she has been giving herself the nurturance that she did not receive as a child. Her schema thus changes to include the possibility that she is a nurturing person who can parent herself.

One person realized through a dream interpretation that he was a lovable person and that he did not have to prove this to everyone. Another example is from a colleague who was talking in therapy about whether to have a baby. She had a series of dreams over several weeks about caring for babies. At first she did not know how to do the basics of feeding and bathing a baby, but in each dream she was able to do more and finally was able to take care of a baby. It is interesting to note that during this time, my colleague was not exposed to caring for any babies so it was not actual experience that caused the changes but restructuring her thoughts and views about herself. In all of these cases, insight involved a cognitive–experiential shift in the way these people viewed themselves. One could conceptualize most of the changes that occur in verbal therapies as being due to the restructuring of schemata.

The Role of Therapist Interpretation

The most typical way to promote client insight is through therapist interpretation (Hill et al., 1988). Spiegel and Hill (1989) have noted that interpretation is a central technique for producing self-knowledge and change, especially within psychoanalytic theory (Blanck, 1966; Freud, 1914/1953; Fromm-Reichmann, 1950). The way in which interpretation produces changes is by stimulating insight, which can lead to more reality-based feelings and behaviors (Schonbar, 1968). Interpretation can work through bringing unconscious processes into awareness, resolving unconscious conflicts, or allowing the person to reexperience conflicts with parental figures in the transference relationship with the therapist (Levy, 1984).

Because the term "interpretation" is loaded with surplus meanings for many psychotherapists, I want to be sure that readers understand how I use the term. My definition of interpretation is a therapist intervention that goes beyond what the client has overtly stated or recognized, usually presenting a new meaning, reason, or insight for behaviors or feelings that helps clients see things in a new way or from a new framework (Hill, 1985). Note that the definition states nothing about the manner in which the interpretation is delivered. In fact, in this model, I believe that therapists should be tentative and collabora- tive in the manner in which they propose interpretations, so that clients have an opportunity to think about and explore the ideas and propose revisions to interpretations. Thus, I do not believe that therapists should provide clients with a complete and final statement about what their dreams mean, although I recognize that many therapists have this connotation of interpretation.

Likewise, Natterson (1993), a psychoanalytic therapist, indicated that when a therapist who wants to exert power over a dreamer offers a shocking interpretation of a dream, it usually has an antitherapeutic effect. Such an interpretation discourages the dreamer from creating and sharing his or her dream. Natterson noted that a therapist is not a police detective waiting to discover the dreamer's fatal flaw and then leaping interpretively upon the unsuspecting patient. Reik (1935) simi- larly emphasized the deep, collaborative nature of the therapeutic encounter and suggested that insights should come as a surprise to both the analysand and the analyst.

GUIDELINES FOR IMPLEMENTING
THE INSIGHT STAGE

Before proceeding, I want to emphasize again that interpretations need to be done as a collaborative effort between therapists and clients based on a good working alliance. Therapists do not necessarily have the correct interpretation but rather can offer tentative ideas and chal- lenges for the client to think about. Clients have the keys to their own dreams, with therapists trying to facilitate clients in their quest to solve the puzzle of what dreams are all about. The ideal process is one in which both offer possible interpretations, with clients being the final arbiters of what does and does not fit. Thus, therapists and clients collaboratively engage in the hermeneutic task of constructing meaning out of dreams.

Introducing the Insight Stage

One way of beginning this stage is to ask the client something like the following:

> "Now that you have made all these associations and links to waking life, what do you think the dream means for you?"
> "What do you think the message of the dream is for you?"

Alternatively, the therapist can restate the dream by going through and substituting the client's associations to the dream images and the links to waking life and then ask the client what the dream means. For example, one client had a dream:

> *I am standing in a checkout line at a convenience store and feel pressured by the people behind me to hurry up. I am fumbling to get my money out and am panicked because I do not have enough money. Then I find money elsewhere in my purse where I have hidden it away.*

Her dream could be restated by the therapist using the associations that the client had provided during the Exploration Stage:

> *So, to restate the dream by plugging in the associations: You were at a store where people go to get things when they are in a rush and people are often impatient to get what they want and get out. You often worry about not having enough money, so you hide money away in odd places to make sure that you will never run out. In waking life, you are feeling a lot of pressure to keep to a strict schedule in getting through school on time. You are on scholarship and are constantly worried about money. So what do you think this dream tells you about yourself?*

This restatement helped the client begin to explore the meaning of her dream. She decided that the dream was about anxieties about her major in college, her career goals, and her feelings of insecurity.

Throughout this stage, the therapist can use his or her own experience of the client, his or her knowledge of the client's dynamics and past experiences, and his or her own projections, to help the client understand the dream. In contrast to the Exploration Stage, in which the therapist tries to stay as close as possible to the dreamer's experience, the therapist uses his or her own experience in this stage to help clients go beyond what they are already aware of and attain new levels of understanding. Through using his or her own experience, the therapist can challenge defenses and suggest insights that clients might not be able to achieve. The therapist must also be willing to confront discrepancies in the client's report at this point because that often helps clients begin to see where their problems are. Therapists, of course, must always be careful to gauge the client's reaction to make sure that they are not projecting their own issues onto clients with no basis in reality. Therapists must always be willing to back off if they are wrong or if clients are simply not ready to be pushed so much.

For example, a student in a dream seminar told a dream in which she was a therapist in a mental hospital and then gradually, without really intending to, she became a patient in the hospital. None of her associations had to do with commitment, but because we all knew about her general passivity, we questioned her about whether the dream might have been related to her ambivalence about getting help for herself and in committing herself to relationships and to her education. She agreed with this interpretation and immediately used it to begin exploring what was going on in her life. Had we not known her general issues, we might not have been able to help her piece together these issues in her life with what arose in the dream.

Therapists' ability to take an objective but supportive stance can help clients see new aspects of dreams that they may not have been able to see on their own. Often clients get blocked in trying to go beyond the dream images and put them together in a meaningful way. Therapists thus can often help clients gain new perspectives on their dreams.

Levels of Dream Interpretation

Dreams can be understood at different levels because the dream reflects a variety of issues for the dreamer that are all located within the same schema or related schemata. Using the analogy of an onion, we can keep peeling back the layers to determine how one's reaction to the waking events were influenced by multitudes of past experiences. Dreamers can find valuable information about themselves at each of the levels, although they may not always be interested, willing, or psychologically able to engage in archeological digs to determine all of the roots of dreams. As an example, a dream about a prisoner passively serving a prison term could relate to a waking issue of a lack of assertiveness with a boss; it could also relate to an internal issue over passivity versus activity; it could reflect problems in relationships with one's peers; it could have its origins in childhood relationships with parents. Any given dream probably has a number of valid interpretations because people are complicated creatures with every current feeling being multideter-mined from many past experiences.

Jungian therapists (Faraday, 1974; Johnson, 1986; Jung, 1974) offer a somewhat similar description of the levels of dream interpreta-tion in their distinction between the objective and subjective levels of interpretation. The objective level relates to current waking reality, such that the dream is about something that is happening in waking life. At the subjective level, the dream represents deeper issues for the person. In the present model, we have extended these from two to four levels of interpretation: as an experience in and of itself, as a reaction to waking events, as a reflection of past memories, and as parts of oneself.

Dream Experience

In dreams, people do things that they ordinarily would not do. Reflecting on these actions in dreams offers clients the opportunity to see what their feelings and reactions are in these situations. Thus, rather than considering the dream to be representative of something else, it is considered as an experience that is important in and of itself. For example, a client who has a dream about quitting his job could be helped to think about what that experience was like for him. The therapist could ask him what he learned about himself as a person who would quit his job. By thinking about quitting his job in the dream, the client could come to a clearer sense of whether that was something he wanted to do. A client with a dream about flying could be helped to think about what kind of person she would be if she could fly. If a man dreams of having a wild affair after his wife dies, the therapist can help the client think about what that possibility means for him personally—what new things can he learn about himself knowing that he is the type of person who would have a wild affair? If a person dreams about killing his parents, examining the dream at this level presents an opportunity for that person to learn something about the depth of his feelings. Thus, by examining this level, clients can learn more about who they are as people and about the depths of their wishes, desires, fears, doubts, and feelings.

In their phenomenological model, Craig and Walsh (1993) similarly suggested that dreams can be understood as important phenomena in and of themselves without considering them as reflections of something else. From this perspective, therapists need to help people understand how they experienced situations presented in dreams.

Relation to Current Waking Events

Given that dreams reflect and often continue waking thoughts without the influence of external cues present during waking life (see Chapter 2 review), dreams can be used to help clients understand how they feel about current events in waking life. Using the previous example of the dream in which a man was having a wild affair after his wife died, we might discover that the dream was triggered by the client's feelings of repressed jealousy about his wife talking to another man at a party. By examining the dream, the therapist can help the client explore his anger at his wife for a situation that actually occurred.

At this level, the dream tells dreamers something about their current life situations. Probably all of us have experienced dreaming about actual events that have taken place. While I was working on this book, I had many dreams about writing sections of the book. Students studying for tests often dream about taking the test. Waitresses dream about waiting on tables and dealing with customers. We often keep on working at night in our dreams. Thus, dreams often relate very directly to specific events in one's life.

Reality dreams might also be about interpersonal issues in one's daily life. Thus, a dream about a friend being angry at you might signal that you have interpersonal problems with that person. You may have partially noticed his or her nonverbal behavior but failed to ask about it. Or you may not have noticed the behaviors because you did not want the person to react that way. Dreams often cue us into feelings or issues that we do not have time to think about or do not allow ourselves to think about when awake.

It seems appropriate to interpret some dreams at only the level of the waking event because they mimic real life so closely. For example, a male college student dreamed that he was at a wedding banquet and saw an old girlfriend across the room. In the dream, he sat down and talked with his old girlfriend. His associations were all about how much he missed his old girlfriend and how much he wanted to reconcile with her, even though he was reluctant to call her because he did not want to admit that he was at fault in a fight that they had had over a year ago. He preferred the idea of running into her without his having to initiate the contact. He identified the trigger as an invitation to a wedding. The dream did not contain much metaphor or symbolism, but rather seemed similar to his waking fantasies. This dreamer was not very introspective and had no desire to delve into deeper aspects of his personality, so staying with the level of his wishes for this event to occur in waking life and how he could make that happen were all we were able to pursue. Talking about the dream, however, helped him clarify his feelings about his old girlfriend and his need to act on his feelings.

In the past, dreams have been used to diagnose illnesses and foretell the future (Kramer, 1982). For example, one therapist told of a woman who dreamed she had an orange growing under her arm. The therapist advised this woman to go to the doctor, who diagnosed the beginnings of a tumor under her arm. Faraday (1974) indicated that if she dreamed that the brakes were failing on her car, it might mean that something actually was wrong with the brakes. She might have subliminally or subconsciously picked up clues during the day about her failing brakes, but only had time to process this information during her dreams.

Relation to Past Memories

Perhaps one of the most typical ways of examining one's present reactions is to examine past memories. Present behavior is often strongly influenced by past experiences. Thus, we may have a strong reaction to someone in the present because of events that occurred in the past. Dreams can also be interpreted by helping the dreamer understand his or her reaction to the waking event in relation to past memories. Continuing the example of the dream of a man having a wild affair after his wife died, the man's jealousy about his wife's flirting might have been because of past situations in which he felt displaced by a younger sibling. Because the waking event triggers thoughts, feelings, and memories stored in schemata, dreams can be interpreted as relating directly to people or events in one's past. Of course, much of psychodynamic therapy involves examining current reactions in relation to past memories (i.e., transference).

As an example, a student presented a dream for a class demonstration in which her therapist refused to see her in a private office but instead conducted their therapy session in the middle of a busy reception area. During the middle of the session, the dreamer went to the bathroom and discovered a dead body of a woman in a bathtub. She knew intuitively in the dream that the woman had been murdered by her (the dreamer's) therapist. During her associations, she discussed difficulties she was having trusting her therapist. Thus, her dream clearly related to issues that were going on in her current life. However, while she was associating to the blood in the bathtub, she had a sudden vivid memory of her father falling in the shower when she was young and her seeing his blood all over the bathroom. This memory led us to explore how her trust issues in therapy might be related to her relationship with her parents, particularly her father.

Parts of Self

One could view the images in dreams as representing parts of the dreamer, given that the dreamer has identified with and introjected parts of significant others into him- or herself. Psychoanalytic theorists (e.g., Greenson, 1967) have discussed the construct of projective identification, where unresolved historical conflicts are projected onto current signifi- cant others, who then play out the part and project their own issues. So dreams reveal a constant cycling of past issues onto current experiences that are played out in terms of past issues. One could thus say that one's inner conflicts are projected onto other people or objects in the dream. Perls (1969) suggested that, "All the different parts of the dream are yourself, a projection of yourself" (p. 69). Similarly, Jungians believed that all parts of the dream are parts of oneself, in that each person has many parts (e.g., persona, anima or animus, shadow, trickster, etc.). From this perspective, the parts of the dream in the previous example could all represent parts of the man; perhaps one part of him wants to have a wild affair whereas another part of him is dying from lack of attention.

By imagining that specific dream elements represent parts of ourselves, we can begin to explore the many facets of our schemata (i.e., in our memories). An example is a dream a woman reported in which her husband was having an affair with another woman. In terms of waking life, the woman indicated that her husband was very faithful and that she knew he would, in fact, never have an affair. So we explored what part of her was like her husband, given that perhaps her "dream husband" represented a part of her. Her husband was used as a metaphor in the dream for the feelings inside her. She realized that the dream was indeed about her own issues regarding commitment and fidelity.

Another example is a dream that a graduate student had of being on a bus. In the dream, a young boy jumps off the bus and runs away. The dreamer's sister chases the young boy but can never catch him. The dreamer stops the driverless bus and then gets off and catches the boy. The dreamer was asked to imagine about what parts of him were like the young boy, his sister, and the driverless bus. Each of these parts fit different aspects of the dreamer—his wanting to run away like the young boy, being like his sister and wanting to fix everything, feeling out of control like the driverless bus, and being the one to put the brakes on when things get out of control. By thinking about the dream as representing different parts of himself, the dreamer was able have more insight into different parts of his personality.

Choosing between Levels

Determining which level to pursue is often complicated. The choice requires a clinical decision about what issues currently are most impor- tant. As an example, a client presented a dream in which she was pursued by a large, ferocious tiger. She attempted to jump higher and higher to get away from it, but it finally caught her and grabbed her. The client's associations were that the images were sexual, and she thought the dream may have been indicative of childhood sexual abuse.

She knew she had been physically and emotionally abused as a child but had no memories of sexual abuse. When asked about recent events, the client revealed that on the day prior to the dream she had been in a rage at her boss for an issue that involved neglecting her needs. Previous issues with the boss tended to reflect unresolved conflicts with her mother who was extremely self-centered and demanding of the client. The therapist had to choose between exploring the possible sexual abuse even though the client had no substantiating memories or to pursue the relevant immediate connection of her rage at her boss, which of course would also eventually lead back to old issues. In this case, the therapist chose to focus on the immediate pressing issue of anger, which the client always wanted to "stay above." The therapist had to balance neither minimizing nor emphasizing the sexual abuse issues with gently helping the client to look at her anger in the immediate situation and how it was related to past, unresolved issues.

To get to the deeper levels of interpretation, therapists have to determine whether clients are ready. Therapists can do this by offering tentative questions about associations of images to past significant others, or they can speculate about whether reactions to current events are related to past events. Therapists have to walk a fine line between being gentle with clients and challenging their defenses so that they can learn more about themselves. Again, if a collaborative alliance has been established, therapists can support clients when they get into difficult issues and ask clients to tell them if they are not willing to go further.

Each of these four levels of interpretation can provide valuable information for the dreamer. Indeed, clients can learn a lot about themselves from using other methods of dream interpretation (e.g., Freudian, Jungian, Adlerian, Gestalt). We do not have any empirical evidence that any level or method is necessarily any more valid than any other (see Chapter 12 for a review of the research). Some dreams provide a wealth of material for many sessions. Because dreams mean many different things, dreamers can continue to learn things about themselves through several sessions of interpretation. Trying out the various levels of interpretation can lead dreamers to examine different aspects of their lives.

If clients are very literal and have a hard time examining themselves on a deeper level, they may not be willing or able to go beyond looking at the dream as a reflection of waking events. It is important for therapists to match their interventions to what clients can handle.

Accuracy of Interpretation

Determining the accuracy of the interpretation is probably not possible. As with other types of interpretations in therapy, perhaps the criterion should be on utility rather than accuracy (Frank & Frank, 1991; Liebert & Spiegler, 1987). Reid and Finesinger (1952) suggested that insight does not need to be "true" but merely needs to be believed to have a therapeutic effect. Furthermore, Reid and Finesinger thought that the important factor is not the truth per se but rather the relevance of the interpretation, psychologically, to the client's problems. I am not suggesting that therapists should ignore the truth, but rather that one can never know for sure if an insight is accurate. If an interpretation helps a client understand some new aspects of him- or herself and leads to some action, then it has been helpful. Because the client is encouraged in this model to construct the insight, there is minimal danger of imposing an inaccurate interpretation from outside.

We can, however, discuss criteria for determining whether an interpretation is helpful for a client. When an interpretation is helpful, the client typically has a sense of "Aha," of learning something that fits or "clicks," and feels that things make sense in a new way. It is important that this feeling comes from the client rather than from the therapist. In addition, clients generally have a feeling of energy and excitement when they are on the right track in terms of understanding the dream.

Another important issue is that the interpretation needs to fit together as many pieces of the dream as possible. Often in a first attempt at interpreting a dream, the client will leave out significant pieces. For example, in a dream that a graduate student presented about being in a prison and seeing his brother there, he first interpreted the dream as reflecting his waking concerns about working in the prison. But that interpretation did not incorporate the contemptuous feelings that he had to all the prisoners except his brother, who he thought had been imprisoned unfairly, nor did it capture the presence of cartoon characters who were on the bunk above his brother. We had to struggle further to discover a more complete interpretation.

Having Clients Summarize Major Learnings

Once some understanding of an interpretation is reached, it is sometimes useful for the therapist to ask the dreamer to summarize the meaning of the dream in one or two sentences. Summarizing helps dreamers consolidate what they have learned and put it in their own language. For example, when I asked her to summarize what she had learned, one client said that the dream revealed that she had concerns about whether she wanted an exclusive relationship with her boyfriend. Thus, she was able to take the work we had done and put it in a phrase that she could take out with her. Articulating this concern hopefully enabled her to continue thinking about the issue.

Sometimes in hearing the summary, therapists become aware that clients have not heard, found important, or integrated all that was discussed. In the last example, the client focused only on the relationship issues and omitted summarizing the work we had done on her self-esteem issues. By confronting her with this omission, we were able to look at her reluctance to work on her self-esteem issues.

Often, beginning to put the dream together causes the therapist to realize that some parts of the dream remain vague because they were not explored enough. Hence, the therapist may need to elicit further associations from the client about images of the dream. Cycling between the first two stages is common as new issues emerge in the work.

THERAPIST TECHNIQUES
THAT FACILITATE INSIGHT

Interpretation

Probably the most important (though not necessarily the most frequent) therapist intervention in this stage is interpretation. Interpretations go beyond what the client has overtly stated or recognized; present a new meaning, reason, or explanation for behaviors, feelings, or thoughts; establish connections between statements or events; point out patterns or themes; point out defenses, resistances, or transference; relate present events to past events; or give a new framework to feelings, behaviors, and problems (Hill, 1985). Research generally indicates that interpretations should be of moderate depth (i.e., just beyond the client's current level of awareness) and tailored specifically to the client's interpersonal difficulties (see review in Hill, 1992). Examples are as follows:

"I wonder if you're having fears of death because your mother is sick."

"Perhaps you dreamed about your brother using drugs because you still have fears that you will slip back into drug use."

Not every dream will yield an immediate interpretation, nor will clients agree with every interpretation offered by therapists. If an interpretation cannot be reached readily, it is better not to force it but to wait until the client brings in another dream to clarify the issues. A series of dreams often provides a better understanding of the underlying conflict or problem than does a single dream (Hall, 1947; Urbina, 1981).

Therapists need to be careful not to force their own interpretations on clients because this stifles the exploration process and makes it difficult for clients to take responsibility for their dreams (Delaney, 1993). Therapists should not ignore their hunches about the meaning of dreams but should be willing to set them aside in case they are wrong or the client is not ready to hear them.

Confrontation

Confrontations point out discrepancies or contradictions of which the client is unaware, and they challenge the client to explain or resolve the discrepancy (Hill, 1985). Confrontations require clients to stretch beyond what they currently believe and to think about their assumptions. Confrontations can be very useful in this stage to help clients realize that they are avoiding or missing crucial issues and are often necessary to break through defenses. Although very little is known empirically about the best manner for delivering confrontations, I think it is safe to say that the most effective interpretations are probably done tentatively and in a supportive, nonhostile manner. For example, the therapist might say the following:

> "I wonder if you aware that even though you say you want to understand the possible connection between your image of a vicious monster and your mother, every time I bring it up you get quiet and don't say anything."
> "Even though you say that everything seems fine right now in your life, your dream has a lot of danger and a sense of foreboding. I wonder how that fits together for you?"

In my experience, beginning therapists are often hesitant to use confrontations because they fear that they are intruding on the client's privacy. However, if the therapist does not confront the client's maladaptive beliefs, it will be difficult for the client to change. The challenge to the therapist is to present the confrontation in a way that the client can hear and yet feel supported.

Facilitative Interventions

As in the Exploration Stage, the majority of therapist interventions during the Insight Stage probably will be open-ended questions ("What do you think the dream means?"), reflections of feelings ("It sounds like it really hurts when you think about your mother not being there for you"), and minimal encouragers ("Mm hmm," nonverbal responsiveness). Thus, after therapists interpret or confront, they need to support clients and facilitate the exploration of the new materials.

Rarely Used Interventions

As in the Exploration Stage, therapists will seldom probe for what clients would like to do differently or give direct advice about what clients could do differently outside the therapy session. These interventions are saved for the Action Stage when therapists have more of a foundation of what dreams mean to clients.

EXTENDED EXAMPLE: FLUNKING A COURSE

This session was the third of 12 sessions of a successful case conducted within the context of brief individual therapy for the Diemer et al. (1996) study. The client was a 30-year-old married woman with a high school education and no children. She was just starting her own decorating business after working for someone else for several years. Her presenting problems were bouts of depression over starting her own business and concerns about how to relate to people with whom she worked. Her therapist was an experienced, 43-year-old, female doctoral student with a humanistic/psychodynamic theoretical orientation.

The therapist and client worked for about 30 minutes on the Exploration Stage exploring each of the images in the dream. This example picks up where the therapist introduced the Insight Stage. The transcript has been edited to make it shorter and easier to read, but the content has not been altered. C stands for client and T stands for therapist in the transcript. The client and therapist both read the transcript of this session and gave consent for it to be used in the book.

The Dream

I signed up for two courses. I could never get to the room on time for one of them because I couldn't find the room. If I did find it, I got there way too late. As a result, I had to drop out of that class. But I was taking one other class, and I thought I did very well in that course. I was in a room with a bunch of people, and we were getting together a project. The opposing team is on the other side of the hallway and it's sort of separated by glass partitions. But their door is ajar a little bit, so I'm looking, trying to peer in to see what they're up to and if we're going to be able to beat them. I saw a little bit and didn't get very good vibes from that room. My ex-boss was in there. I leave that room and walk over to get my grades from the course that I was taking. So I'm walking across campus thinking, "Wow, it's too bad I had to drop out of that course." I didn't understand why I could not find the room in time and felt down on myself that I had to drop out. I walk up to the door that has the grades and see that I failed. I was really shocked because I thought I did really well in the course. I leave and start running and running and then I'm jumping over this stone wall. I'm thinking, "Why did I do badly in

*a course that I thought that I passed?" Then I get back to the room
where the people are and explain to them, "I can't believe this, I
thought I did really well, I didn't do well." They also are shocked by
the whole situation because they thought I was doing well too.*

T: Let's go through the dream and reframe the dream from the associations. You talk about being in a closed-in, confined, stagnant area
and you can't find your way. You're lost, confused, kind of out of touch
with things. You also associated the room to comraderie, working on a
project together. I asked you about being late to a class, which again
brought up confusion, and irresponsibility, child-like, missing out on
something. Dropping the class is giving up, giving in to the confusion,
and not being able to ask for help or to say that you're lost. Between the
two rooms, there's this competition which you feel is pressure and
stress. There's this need to achieve, but if you do achieve, that's empow-
ering but the pressure's also very hard on you. Then when you look
through this glass partition, it's a block, a protection, but it's a false
sense of protection. You can kind of see through it, but it's a false
separation. In the dream, the glass was separating where you used to
be from where you are now. I'm wondering what that false separation
or protection might be between the two rooms?

C: I think because I'm away from where I used to work, but I'm still
connected because she owes us a lot of money. She's trying to intimidate
us legally not to pursue getting that money. So that's what it is. I feel
protected now that I'm away from it, but it's a false protection, a false
block, because I still have that connection with her through the money
thing.

T: All right, there's a hallway that you said is another street, a
separation, a thoroughfare, where you can enter and exit, and there's a
door that you said is an opening and entrance or escape. When the door
is ajar, it's kind of like you're peeping into, you're prying, nosy, curious,
interested in something. You see a little bit, but then you get these bad
vibes, so you're curious about what's going on in there. You want to look,
but when you do get a look, you pick up these bad vibes, which you
associated to as negative, disharmonious, their project's not as good as
yours. There's no creativity there. When you peep into the store, you
see your ex-boss and that creates tenseness. When you think of her, you
think of someone being vain, fake, out for money, everything's money,
and also a threat. Is there anyone in your life right now that would
maybe be like your ex-boss?

C: My brother Jack is really nutso lately. He's a lot like that right now.
He's having problems. I had a blowout with him a couple weeks ago. We
had a family gathering about what we were going to do about Dad. We're
going to sell the house, so we have to come up with some way to find a
house and who's going to be responsible for that home. Every time I

opened my mouth to say something, he'd say "Oh, pipe down." Finally, I got up right in his face and said, "If you say that to me one more time, I don't know what I'm going to do, but you're just pissing me off, this is just being downright rude." He's the only one I can think of that I have any kind of conflict with besides my ex-boss. Since then he hasn't called me, and I haven't called him, and he hasn't come over to see the new showroom or anything.

T: So that relationship is kind of estranged right now.

C: Mm hmm, we had a problem last summer. We had a really bad fight. When I tried to call him to make amends, he said he'd only talk to me with a psychologist. I agreed with that, thinking it would help him, so we went. But I've had problems with him in the past, so he might have something to do with this dream.

T: Then when you leave that area, and you associated leaving with being adventurous, expecting, kind of wondering what you're going to find there. And also abandonment, separation, and sadness . . .

C: That's exactly how I felt when I left my old job. The day I gave my notice, she fired me because she found out. I cried, and she gave me a hug and everything. She was being totally fake because 2 weeks later she was being really nasty. But I did feel sad leaving there because I had been there for so many years. I knew her husband, and he was really wonderful. He got that business going really well, and I really liked him. I told her it felt like I was losing my best friend almost because I had been there for so many years and it's been so good to me. She gave me a hug and then turned around and got her lawyer after us and wouldn't pay us our money and slandered me and my partner to other people. It was awful.

T: She's still having an effect on you in some way.

C: Yeah.

T: If you were to summarize this dream for yourself in a sentence or two, the meaning that you got from the dream, how would you do that?

C: It's definitely directly related to how I'm feeling lately. It's everything that's been happening in a nutshell. The meaning I get is that my life right now is sort of in a turmoil and that I need to take steps to make myself feel better about it. I think it's getting to the real deep meaning of my sense of confusion lately of being out of touch with myself and not ever really having felt like I got help to get rid of that sense of confusion. Even though I've always been really good at whatever I do, I always have this real bad insecurity problem, always fearing that I'm not going to do well when I know darn well that I'm capable of it. My two brothers are the real reason I feel insecure and blame myself for a lot. They put us through a lot of emotional abuse when we were growing up, very similar to the emotional abuse that my ex-boss generated.

T: It sounds like it's still happening, him putting you down and telling you to be quiet and not to talk.

C: Right, I feel that way when I speak with him. I feel that way in social situations. I feel like what I have to say is not as important as what other people have to say or that people don't really care if I show up or not.

T: Like the class, you were probably registered but no one looked for you, so it didn't matter that you didn't get there.

C: Yeah.

Commentary

This client brought in a recurrent dream of flunking a class. The therapist first spent about half an hour having the client tell the dream, associate to each of the major images, and then link these associations to waking life. In introducing the Insight Stage, the therapist summarized the associations and then asked the client about the meaning of the dream. The client talked about her current job situation and linked her difficulties with her previous boss to abuse by her brother. The therapist ended the Insight Stage by asking the client to summarize what she had learned, with the client confirming that the dream was about her current life situation but had links to childhood. Thus, the therapist focused primarily on the second and third levels of interpretation, relating the dream to waking life and to past memories. She did not examine the dream as an experience in and of itself nor did she focus on the parts of the dream being parts of the dreamer.

One feature that stands out in the example is that the therapist did not give an interpretation to the client. Rather, they worked together to understand what the dream was about for the client. They clearly had a good relationship, with mutual trust and respect. The therapist followed the dream interpretation model closely, but at no point did the process seem rigid or stilted. In fact, the therapist was very comfortable with the approach because it fit her gentle, supportive, client-centered style. This example also illustrates how therapists recycle back through associations and links to waking life while they are in the Insight Stage. The remainder of this session is continued in the next chapter.

SUMMARY

The Insight Stage is the place to try to put together what the client and therapist together have learned about the dream. The raw material for this stage is the initial dream, the associations to the images, the emotional arousal attached to the images, and the links of the images to waking life. Additionally, the therapist at this point brings in his or her experience of the dreamer, his or her knowledge about the dreamer's dynamics and past experiences, and his or her own projections, all of which dreamers would have no access to when trying to interpret dreams on their own. The dream can be understood at many different levels, ranging from the dream experience, to the waking events, to memories of previous events, and to parts of oneself. Insight involves changes in schemata as people come to restructure their thoughts and understandings of themselves. As some parts of the dream are understood better, it is typical for therapists and clients to return to explore other parts of the dream more thoroughly, so there is some interplay between the stages of exploration and insight.

CHAPTER SEVEN

Action Stage

EXPLORATION AND INSIGHT should lead directly to action so that clients have a greater awareness of what they would like to change in their lives. Reid and Finesinger (1952) noted that, unless self-knowledge gained from insight helps clients change their emotional attitudes toward the past and future, insight can be just another sad variation on the theme of failure. On the other hand, action without insight is often misdirected and does not remedy the problem because it is based on faulty assumptions. Thus, insight and action both seem to me to be necessary components of the change process. Table 7.1 shows the goals of the Action Stage, the tasks to be accomplished, the most frequently used and rarely used therapist techniques, and the desired therapist manner.

Many theorists (e.g., Gendlin, 1986; L. S. Greenberg & Safran, 1987) have noted that once emotions are experienced, an action tendency emerges. Similarly, some analysts (Applebaum, 1973; Reid & Finesinger, 1952) have assumed that insight leads directly to change. And indeed, some clients do change spontaneously after achieving insight. For example, one client dreamed that she was getting married but was wearing a black see-through dress to her wedding. After associating to weddings and black dresses, she came to understand that the dream was about her anxiety about getting married. As she talked about her awareness of this anxiety, she also realized that she needed to be careful about how she dressed in waking life so that she did not look so seductive. Thus, her newfound insight led directly to her thinking about what she needed to do differently in her waking life.

However, insight does not automatically trigger new behavior in *all* clients (see also Orlinsky & Howard, 1986; Spiegel & Hill, 1989). Some clients need to be helped to make changes. They cannot get beyond insight to figuring out what to do differently on their own. In effect, they get stuck in the Insight Stage and need the impetus to move on to the next stage. Others may be motivated to change things in their lives but do not have the necessary skills in their repertoire. These clients need to be taught skills (e.g., appropriate eye contact, assertiveness, relaxation) or be given feedback about inappropriate behaviors (e.g., constantly putting oneself down, incessant giggling). Therapists can assist clients in taking action by helping them determine what they would like to do differently on the basis of their new understanding of their dreams.

The foundation for action is the change in the schemata that occurred in the Insight Stage. Action should follow from how the client has come to reconceptualize the problem for him- or herself. Taking action helps consolidate the changes in the schemata gained through the Insight Stage. New connections are strengthened through repeated practice, whereas old connections are weakened. Without the action, the insights would remain as weak connections and would undoubtedly deteriorate without use. Thus, action seems to be essential to ensure that change takes place.

I believe that the goal of all therapy is to help clients change their thoughts, feelings, and/or actions. Similarly, the goal of dream interpretation is to enable clients to make changes in thinking and in their lives. Thus, the Action Stage is very important and should not be overlooked.

TABLE 7.1. Outline of the Action Stage

I. Goals
- A. Use data from Exploration and Insight Stages to facilitate changes in client's life.
- B. Use action to consolidate changes in client's schemata
- C. Maintain the therapeutic alliance

II. Tasks
- A. Choose one or more types of action.
    1. Changing the dream
        a. In fantasy
        b. While dreaming
    2. Continued work on the dream
    3. Behavioral or life changes
- B. Have client summarize what he or she learned from the dream.

III. Therapist techniques
- A. Frequently used techniques: Open-ended questions, minimal encouragers, reflection of feelings, direct guidance, information
- B. Less frequently used techniques: Interpretation

IV. Therapist manner
- A. Collaborative
- B. Facilitative

The following various types of action are possible, depending on the therapist's judgment about what would be most clinically useful:

- Changing the dream
- Continued work on the dream
- Behavioral or life changes

CHANGING THE DREAM

Changing the Dream in Fantasy

The most natural and easiest step after the Insight Stage is to ask the client how he or she would like to change the dream in fantasy. In asking a client to change the outcome of the dream, therapists might suggest that he or she remove any constraints and finish the dream in a different way. One way to phrase this query is to say, "If you could change the dream in any way that you wished, what is your fantasy of how would you like to change it?"

With a recurrent dream of being rejected by a boy whom she had liked during childhood, a dreamer was asked to say how she would like to have the dream turn out in her fantasy. She responded that she would like to approach the boy rather than wait for him to notice her. We then talked about how she could approach the boy in such a way as to make acceptance more likely. In another example of a recurrent dream about being chased by a big bear, the dreamer said she would like to chase the bear instead of having it chase her. These examples illustrate that changing the dream can be fun and playful, often giving dreamers a sense of empowerment that dreams are their own creations and they can change dreams if they wish.

Sometimes clients get stuck trying to think of ways to change dreams. Perhaps they feel overwhelmed by the emotions and feel helpless to change even their fantasies. In such cases, the therapist might say what his or her fantasy would be. For example, the therapist might say, "If it were my dream, I would want to make up with my friend after the fight. How would that feel for you?"

Noting what clients choose to change in their dreams can be very revealing. For example, in the dream of a woman observing her dead body being carried down the stairs by several anonymous, respectful men, the woman indicated that what she would change is having the men be more clear so that she would know who they were and what they were thinking. It was very revealing that she did not change being dead and observing herself rather than being in her body. Challenging her about this omission led to further exploration of what was going on for her.

Changing the Dream While Dreaming

Clients who have troubling dreams or nightmares (e.g., replays of sexual abuse, war traumas, natural disasters) need to have ways of coping with the bad dreams during the night when they cannot sleep or when they are so terrified that they do not want to return to sleep. They need to gain a sense of control, a sense that they are not powerless in the grips of the dream.

Cartwright and Lamberg (1992) present a crisis method for teaching clients to deal with particularly bad dreams. Their RISC model teaches clients to *recognize* bad dreams, *identify* what it is about the dream that makes the person feel bad, *stop* the dream, and *change* the dream dimensions from negative to positive. Cartwright and Lamberg noted that, rather than changing the waking situation and hoping that changes in dreams will follow, one can change the dream and changes in waking life will follow. They noted that it is often easier to change the dream than to change the waking situation and that changing the dream can provide dreamers with a sense of empowerment. This RISC method is particularly valuable when clients are feeling like helpless victims, because it gives them a way to feel some control over their lives. Going back to sleep and changing the outcome of the dream is a form of lucid dreaming (Gackenbach & Bosveld, 1989; LaBerge, 1985), in which the dreamer becomes aware that he or she is dreaming and takes control of the dream. They report that clients can learn to stop their bad dreams after just a few sessions. I recommend that therapists try this method. Once the client has gained some control over the bad dreams, it is easier to go back and try to understand what caused the dreams to occur.

When my children awoke with nightmares (which are typical among young children), I sometimes suggested that they go back to sleep and beat up the monster. Being able to fight the monster helped them to feel powerful and not to feel as frightened. Other times I have suggested that they go back and make friends with the monster. These suggestions helped my children go back to sleep and not feel so helpless—they had skills they could use to deal with the monster. Similarly, the client who had the dream about the vicious tiger attacking her could learn to embrace the tiger as a part of herself, which could instigate further changes in her schemata about power and victimization.

Redoing the end of a dream, either in fantasy or during the dream, can lead one to feel a sense of mastery over the dream, over one's view of self, and over one's life. By realizing that they are not just passive recipients of their dreams but rather are active players in the production of dreams, people can learn to take more responsibility for their views of themselves, which are reflected in their dreams and in waking life.

CONTINUED WORK ON THE DREAM

A dream interpretation might raise issues about which a client needs to continue working. Seldom does a client understand a dream completely in a single dream interpretation. There are many layers to the dream that could be explored endlessly. Hence, during this stage the therapist might want to continue work that was started on the dream if it was productive. For example, the therapist might want to help the client work more with issues that came up during the first two stages of the dream interpretation, using some of the suggestions that were given in Chapter 5 on the Exploration Stage (conflict splits, unresolved feelings, dialogues with different parts of the dream, or role playing parts of the dream).

To facilitate continued work on the dream outside of therapy, the therapist might ask the client to go through the dream again using the self-guided manual reprinted at the end of the book. Or the therapist could suggest that the dreamer write about the dream in a journal, continue thinking about associations to particular images, talk with friends about it, or paint the dream. Looking for similarities across a series of dreams might be a way of examining changes in feelings. The main idea here is to keep the dream alive and to continue working on it. As new ideas come up, the client can bring them back to the therapist for more work during the session. In this way, the therapist serves as a coach to help the client begin to work on his or her own outside therapy.

One method for helping clients change their dreams is through active imagination where the dreamer goes in and enacts parts of the dream to learn more about the parts of themselves represented by the dream images (Johnson, 1986). With the client whose dream was about werewolves and vampires, I suggested that he have a dialogue with the werewolves and vampires and discover what they had to say to him. Because we did not have time to do the dialogue within the context of the single session, I suggested that he might want to write the dialogue. He was quite enthusiastic about this idea because he loved to write. Immediately he thought about writing it as a play.

Another possibility would be to work with the client in hypnosis and help him or her reexperience the dream and perhaps imagine a different ending. Hypnosis might be especially helpful with recurrent dreams and nightmares.

Johnson (1986) advocated using rituals as a way of helping dreamers encapsulate what they learned from their dreams and keep the dreams alive. For example, a person who learned that he or she was still hanging on to an old relationship might burn or bury all the things that reminded him or her of that relationship. An example of a more symbolic gesture might be setting a twig in a stream to float away with the current downriver as a representation of letting go of a relationship.

Another example is a person who bought and cared for an African violet to remind herself of a dream in which she forgave her mother (now dead) after a lifetime of bitter fighting with her. Johnson suggests that the ritual be something concrete and feasible, rather than something vague such as thinking about the problem.

I would not suggest that dreamers always need to perform some ritual based on what they learn from the dream. Sometimes either the dreamer is simply not ready to do anything or nothing specific comes to mind. For dreamers who need a sense of closure to their dreams, however, planning a specific ritual can be an excellent way to give clients something concrete and metaphorical to do as a way of reaching some resolution regarding the issues of the dream.

BEHAVIORAL OR LIFE CHANGES

A third type of action is making actual behavioral changes. Much has been written (e.g., Goldfried & Davison, 1994; Watson & Tharp, 1989) about helping clients increase adaptive behaviors (e.g., relaxation, studying behaviors) and decrease maladaptive behaviors (e.g., overeating, inappropriate social behaviors).

Therapists can help dreamers explore what they would like to do differently in their lives based on what they have learned in the dream. Because action does not automatically follow insight, therapists sometimes need to facilitate clients in solidifying their gains through action.

A client with a recurrent dream about flunking out of college (even though she was 40 years old and successful) came to understand that she was terrified about failing because she felt that she would lose her identity if she were not successful. She was taught time management skills to help her deal with practical problems. Furthermore, because identity issues were also a big part of the problem, she and the therapist decided to work on identity issues in subsequent therapy.

A client with a dream about eating so much that she exploded decided that she needed to get some control over her eating behavior. The therapist suggested specific exercise and weight control programs. The client chose those parts of the programs that she liked best. She decided to start exercising a few minutes a day. She also decided to eat more moderately, but being aware of how poorly she did when she deprived herself of all sweets, she decided to allow herself one treat each day. After the client began to get her eating and exercising under control, the therapist helped the client think about the role of food in her life. She realized that she often ate when she was angry at people, so they set up an assertiveness training program. Thus, the client chose moderate, realistic goals that she was able to do and made just a few changes at a time.

A client whose dream revealed that he was unhappy in his current job was helped to think about his vocational identity. He decided that he wanted a different kind of job, so he and the therapist talked about how he would go about quitting his current job and also worked on job-hunting strategies.

Sometimes the action that the dreamer decides he or she needs to take is to *not* act in certain ways. For example, one student realized through her dream that her friends all got angry at her because she tried to take control of all situations. She realized that she had to let go and let others make their own mistakes. Not playing the rescuer and not being in control was a difficult task for this woman. Similarly, some people need to learn to accept unpleasant feelings (e.g., depression, guilt) without fighting them. Talking about such action steps can lead to further changes in beliefs.

Change rarely is simple and often requires extensive examination of what clients really want to do. Much of therapy in this stage involves helping clients clarify their values and feelings about different options. However, once clients make decisions about what changes they want to make, they often need specific help in going about making those changes. Thus, therapists need to be prepared with specific knowledge of different behavior change techniques, such as assertiveness training, relaxation training, self-control strategies, job-hunting skills, and communication skills training. It is probably best to work on one problem at a time with limited goals rather than trying to change everything immediately. More information on specific strategies for behavior change can be found in several excellent sources (Alberti & Emmons, 1974; Burns, 1980; Goldfried & Davidson, 1994; Watson & Tharp, 1989).

Many clients are not ready for action during the first dream interpretation. Gauging readiness is important prior to thinking about action. Some clients might say that they want to change, but when it comes down to setting up an action plan they are unwilling to plan anything. Therapists might want to step back at this point and determine if clients are getting some kind of secondary gains out of not changing. For example, a passive client might say that he wants to change but in fact might be getting reinforcement from his wife for being passive. Therapists need to help people decide whether they do in fact want to change and perhaps upset the whole system of their lives. For very resistant or reactant clients, the action that therapists might suggest would be that they "go slow" and make sure not to change too rapidly, a paradoxical technique that can show great empathy for the client (Fisch, Weakland, & Segal, 1982). Therapists need to be willing to back off or change strategies when what they are doing is not working.

Therapists can monitor the effectiveness of their change strategies by examining the dreams that their clients bring in. Evidence (see Chapter 12) indicates that dream content changes over the course of successful therapy, so therapists should expect to see changes in dreams as clients improve (e.g., dreams should have less depressive content as the client becomes less depressed). Dreams might also reveal client dissatisfactions with therapist strategies. For example, a dream that the therapist is pushing her over a cliff might reveal that the client feels a need for more support and less pushiness from the therapist.

THERAPIST TECHNIQUES
THAT FACILITATE ACTION

As in the other stages, the therapist serves as a facilitator in this stage, helping clients discover how they would like to change. Action typically does not work well when therapists decide what clients "should" do and try to get them to do it. When therapists push a particular plan of action on clients, they often encounter resistance from those clients who need to be actively involved in the process.

As with the other two stages, perhaps the most frequent interventions in the Action Stage are open-ended questions (e.g., "What direction does this dream point you in?", "How would you like to change your dream",? "What could you do differently in your life to get that good feeling that you had in your dream?"). And again, reflections of feelings and minimal encouragers are important to help clients clarify how they feel about various action steps.

Therapists also might want to suggest action steps occasionally or provide information to clients about possibilities. Therapists can offer possible action ideas, either collaboratively, such that both therapist and client brainstorm about ideas and choose the best ones, or when clients have no ideas of what they could do differently. For example, in one of my classes, the dreamer had no ideas about action after a long dream interpretation. One of the class members suggested that if the dream were hers, she would want to pamper herself by going on a long vacation. This creative suggestion freed up the dreamer (and the class) to think about other possibilities for taking care of herself. As another example, in a current study we are doing offering single sessions of dream interpretation to volunteer undergraduates, a typical action step that therapists suggest is for students to seek further therapy. One session often is not adequate to deal with all the issues raised in the dream interpretation, so therapists feel a need to offer the availability of services on campus. Similarly, in cases where dreams reveal suicidal thoughts, therapists might want to take a crisis-oriented approach and help clients specifically plan their next few hours and make a contract with them about not committing suicide without calling the therapist first.

Therapists should not get pushy and impose too much action too quickly on clients. If a therapist has become too aggressive or expected too much of a client, he or she can process the interaction by discussing with the client about how he or she felt about the intervention (Cashdan, 1988; Kiesler, 1988). Sometimes it is important to apologize if therapist behavior makes a client feel misunderstood (see Rhodes, Hill, Thompson, & Elliott, 1994). Unfortunately, clients often do not reveal their dissatisfaction with therapist behaviors (Hill, Thompson, Cogar, & Denman, 1993), so therapists have to be very vigilant for signs of dissatisfaction and be willing to ask clients how they are feeling.

In addition, as clients try out new ways of behaving, they sometimes have to go back and try to understand difficulties they have in making changes. As with earlier stages, this might require cycling back to the Exploration and Insight Stages or it might require further therapy.

EXTENDED EXAMPLE: FLUNKING A COURSE

This example is a continuation of the session presented in Chapter 6. C stands for client and T stands for therapist in the transcript. Through the Exploration and Insight Stages, the client came to understand that her dream about flunking a class was related to current concerns about her relationship with her ex-boss and to past concerns about an abusive brother. The Action Stage began after the client summarized what she had learned from the dream.

T: If you could change the dream in any way, how would you make it different?

C: Maybe instead of running back to my friends and family and rehashing the whole thing with them, I should have talked to my professor and asked, "What's the problem, why did I fail, what is it that I did wrong?" But it's hard for me to face someone who is aware of my failure. A good parallel is if I'm working with a client and a mistake occurs, whether it's my fault or whether it's the vendor's fault, it is very hard for me to face them because it makes me feel like their confidence level has just gone way down.

T: So someone else's expectations or their perceptions of you are very important to you.

C: Yeah, I guess that's where I am. I've always had to use the way that people saw me as a gauge because I never had any guidance to help me find it within myself.

T: How are you supposed to know? You never had that modeled for you. What you're doing now is trying to figure that out, which is a very courageous thing to do.

C: I went on a long walk with my sister last weekend. She opened my eyes to a lot about my brother abusing us emotionally and how our parents didn't guide us. It coincided with me working with you. It answered a lot of questions. I'm finding that she experienced it the same way that I did. Talking about it really opened my eyes that I'm not the only one that was affected by it. It really is something that's happened. It's not my imagination.

T: It's not you, right? It's external. It is the circumstances, what has happened.

C: Yeah.

T: How does that feel to know that, to talk with your sister and have that confirmed?

C: It feels really good.

T: Is there anything that you can do as kind of a concrete or symbolic way of owning this dream and doing something to respond to the dream in any way?

C: I thought that I wanted to come here and take a course in business management. It seems to be the logical step. That probably would help a lot. Maybe talk to my partner and not be so afraid that he'll lose confidence in me, because I bet that he has the same fears that I do and he's afraid to tell me.

T: Probably.

C: I guess I should talk to him about it.

T: So how might you go about doing that? Do you want to set a time frame for yourself to do that?

C: It's really hard to talk about anything in the office because we're all together like one big family, so I guess maybe we should go out afterward and talk. We could do that.

T: Something you might want to do before you actually talk is to write down what it is you want to say.

C: That's a good idea, to clear my thoughts up.

T: Yeah. We're coming to a close. How are you feeling about the dream and the work that you did with it today?

C: It made things a lot clearer, it really did.

Commentary

Building on the exploration and insights, the therapist asked the client how she would like to change the dream. The client indicated an awareness that she needed to assert herself in relationships, and then she further explored the role of her family of origin in creating the problem. In response to the therapist's question of what she wanted to change in real life, the client said she might take a course or talk with her partner. The therapist reinforced the idea of talking with her partner and tried to make the idea more concrete by asking about a time for the talk and by suggesting that she write her thoughts down ahead of time. Hence, working with the dream led to a clear identification of a problem that the client had and a commitment to doing something about the problem. Ideally, in future sessions the therapist would follow up on whether the client had talked with her partner and help her with some role plays if she needed modeling and practice on how to do that. The therapist could have followed up more on the client's idea of taking a class in business management at the university as a way to help her counteract the feelings of failure in the dream and as a way to help her handle sticky situations better in the future.

SUMMARY

Based on changes in the schemata from the dream interpretation, direction for change should either appear naturally or be stimulated by the therapist. Insight without action would be sterile. Our ultimate goal as therapists is generally to help clients become less symptomatic, feel better in terms of interpersonal functioning, and become more satisfied with their life situations. Thus, we use what we learn from the dream interpretation to help clients change areas of their lives in directions that make them happier and more productive people.

Many types of change are possible. Changing the ending of the dream, either in fantasy or reality, is often a useful step to empower people to open up to the possibility of change in their lives. Clients can also be encouraged to continue working with their dreams. Incorporating a ritual can help establish in the dreamer's mind that he or she did learn something from the dream, and it can increase motivation to alter the course of one's life. Finally, therapists may need to teach clients new behaviors that were not previously in their behavioral repertoire (e.g., relaxation, assertiveness, study skills, communication skills), or they may need to reinforce clients for using skills that they already possess but are afraid to use. Once again, however, it is important to emphasize that this level of action is appropriate only *after* thorough exploration and insight are done in a very collaborative manner such that the client is ready and asking for help in making behavioral changes.

CHAPTER EIGHT

Therapeutic Issues in Using the Dream Interpretation Model

I N THIS CHAPTER, I discuss a number of therapeutic issues involved in using this model of dream interpretation in the context of ongoing therapy. These issues are the choice of dreams to interpret and with whom to use dream interpretation, introduction of dreams in therapy, use of dreams at specific times in therapy, use of dream images as metaphors later in therapy after the dream interpretation, the impor- tance of the therapeutic relationship, monitoring of client responsive- ness to dream interpretation, the need for flexibility, and counter- transference issues.

CHOICE OF DREAMS TO INTERPRET

Should all dreams be interpreted in therapy? Probably not, especially in a brief therapy. Is every dream important? No—some dreams are trivial, some are fun, some are pure adventure, some are escape. We have several kinds of dreams, some of which probably do not need to be discussed in therapy just as therapists would not ask clients to discuss every thought that comes up during the day.

Should therapists tell clients to write down *all* their dreams so that they can bring them into therapy? Probably not. With unlimited time in therapy, discussion of all dreams could be useful, but given the increasing brevity of treatment, the dreams that most need to be discussed in therapy are the ones that seem salient, important, or troubling to clients. These salient dreams seem to hold the greatest potential for benefiting clients. Hence, the dreams that clients sponta- neously bring up in therapy are the most important. Clients will be most likely, of course, to bring up troubling dreams spontaneously if their therapists let them know that it is valuable to discuss dreams in therapy.

Flowers (1993) cautions, however, that some clients use dreams to avoid working on waking issues. Especially if they know therapists are interested in dreams, clients might present dreams as a defensive maneuver to keep therapists from talking about other important issues. Thus, as with all topics brought up in therapy, therapists need to ask themselves why clients are bringing up dreams to discuss at a particular time.

WHICH CLIENTS ARE APPROPRIATE FOR DREAM INTERPRETATION?

At this point, we have no clear empirical evidence of which clients are most suited for dream interpretation and which are not suited (see review in Chapter 12). Flowers (1993) suggested that the primary indication for using dreams in therapy is client interest. She suggests that men and women of all ages, racial/ethnic backgrounds, educational and occupational levels, and a wide variety of psychiatric diagnoses benefit from working with dreams. A contraindication that Flowers cited is the presence of any thought disorder severe enough to prevent concentration, abstraction, or coherent speech.

From our own research (Diemer et al., 1996), we have found that clients who are cognitively complex, or able to think deeply and elaboratively, benefit most from dream interpretation. From a clinical perspective, such clients are able to associate and play with images. They are interested in dreams and motivated to understand the meaning of the dreams for their lives. In contrast, clients who are very literal and cannot play with images metaphorically are difficult to work with in dream interpretation. Another contraindication to dream interpretation is when clients are unable to distinguish between waking and dreaming states, go into dissociative states, or are frightened by dreamwork.

There are many reasons clients may not want to work with dreams in therapy. Some clients may feel embarrassed by their dreams because they do things in their dreams they would not do in waking life (e.g., unusual sexual or aggressive acts). Some clients may feel frightened by their dreams and want to forget them (e.g., monster dreams). Some clients may feel vulnerable in telling their dreams because they are afraid of what they will reveal about themselves. In addition, the belief that therapists have "the" interpretation of their dreams may make some clients feel vulnerable or out of control. Other clients may feel like dreams are evil and reflect devil possession. Others may feel that dreams are silly and akin to palm reading and astrology, so they might think that talking about dreams in therapy is irrelevant.

Therapists may need to educate such clients about the scientific theory of dream formation and the role of dreams in therapy, perhaps even asking them to read this book. Therapists can suggest (but not promise) that dreams might help clients come to a deeper understanding of themselves and might lead to directions for change. In my experience, educating clients gives them a sense of relief that dreams are personal, understandable, and valuable rather than evil, weird, or silly. Furthermore, the experience of going through a dream interpretation using this model reassures clients that therapists are not going to take over and tell them what the dream means and what to do.

Not everyone remembers their dreams, so dream interpretation is not even possible with all clients. However, innovative programs such as the one developed by Cartwright, Tipton, and Wicklund (1980) could be used to prepare people to use their dreams. Cartwright, Tipton, and Wicklund selected people who were thought to be at risk for dropping out of therapy because of low levels of experiencing. They woke these people during REM sleep and had them tell their dreams. In the morning, they had them think about the meaning of their dreams. People who went through this preparation program benefited more from therapy than those who had not gone through the program. Cartwright, Tipton, and Wicklund also described a pilot preparation program not using the sleep lab. Thus, perhaps people could be trained to recall and then work with their dreams. Instructing clients to keep a journal next to their beds and to write down dreams as soon as they awake could be helpful.

INTRODUCING DREAMS IN THERAPY

Asking clients at the beginning of treatment to bring their dreams into therapy lets them know that therapists believe in the importance of dreams and gives clients permission to talk about dreams. Often, if therapists do not let clients know that they value dreams, clients think that it is not permissible to discuss dreams in therapy. Advising clients about the importance of dreams also lets clients know that it is important to value their own dreams as an avenue to understanding more about themselves. Holding a value for dreams seems to increase recall (Garfield, 1974).

Clients often bring troubling dreams into therapy. If they do so at the beginning of a session, therapists can ask if they would like to work with that dream during that session. If dreams are brought up late in a session, therapists can ask clients to bring the dream up again during the next session so that they can go through all the stages and have enough time to process the dream thoroughly. Therapists can also ask clients to write down their own associations to the dream and bring those in to an upcoming session.

Another issue in choosing a dream to interpret is how recent the dream is. Because dreams from the last few days are generally more vividly remembered, they are easier to interpret than are dreams from the distant past. Moreover, the recent events in the client's life that triggered the dream tend to be clearer and less distorted by events occurring after the dream. Working with old dreams is possible, however, if the dreams are vivid or recurrent and if clients recall what was going on in their lives at the time of the dream. One woman presented a dream that she had when she was 18 months old. We were able to work productively with that dream because the events surrounding the dream were still vivid and traumatic. The woman was able to reexperience the feelings she had at the time of the dream. Dreams from very early life stages may be similar to early recollections (Olson, 1979) and thus are important because they often serve as metaphors for how people view their past. The actual truth of whether the dream occurred at a particular age may not be as important as the belief that the dream (or event) occurred.

USING DREAMS
AT SPECIFIC TIMES IN THERAPY

Some therapists believe that initial dreams are particularly valuable because they condense the important themes that need to be dealt with in therapy. By listening attentively to the first dream, therapists can learn much about clients' problems and fears about the therapy process, as well as hear whether clients have possible solutions for dealing with their problems. As Guntrip (1969) noted, initial dreams can be indicative of attitudes about starting therapy and of feelings that clients have about therapy and therapists in general. We have no empirical evidence about the nature or importance of initial dreams, but it seems reasonable to ask clients about them.

Interpreting a dream during an early session of therapy can also be useful as a way of establishing a relationship with a client. Some clients come into therapy not being able to articulate what is troubling them, and using this structured approach leads them directly to the troubling issues. In addition, the structure can be comforting to clients who are apprehensive about not knowing what to do in therapy. Working on a task together can be a good way of building the relationship.

Dreams can contribute to the process of defining a focus in brief therapy. One client who sought counseling due to a break up with a boyfriend revealed a dream in which she removed her hair and cooked it at her boyfriend's house. As the dream was explored, it became clear that her hair was a symbol of her identity. Consequently, the focus of the treatment shifted to include not only her feelings about the separation from the boyfriend but also her identity issues in the relationship. Dream interpretation seemed to help this client get to her core issues faster than she would have done otherwise.

During the therapy process, a sign that clients are ready or would like to talk about their dreams is when they bring them up. In observing cases of therapy (Hill, 1989), we have noticed that clients do spontaneously bring up dreams, particularly troubling dreams. For example, one client in brief therapy brought up a recurring dream that when she came home, her house had been uprooted and was gone, along with her whole family. Examination of that dream quickly led to discussing her fears of abandonment.

One particularly important time that dreams can be of use in therapy is when there is a therapeutic impasse. A client who comes in with great distress but cannot identify what is troubling him or her or who has a hard time talking about feelings might be asked to bring in a dream. Similarly, if a client is in pain but both the therapist and the client are stuck about how to move forward, asking a client to bring in a dream could help clarify where the client is stuck and indicate where the therapy needs to go. For example, a dream of a little girl huddled in bed might lead to the awareness that the client has unresolved issues about childhood sexual abuse that could be discussed in therapy. Of course, therapists have to be careful not to implant false memories of any kind in clients.

Another time to invite clients to discuss their dreams might be when there are significant transference issues (Hersh & Taub-Bynum, 1985). For example, when clients present dreams that involve the therapist, they may be giving a message that transference issues are important. Clients might have a difficult time bringing up transference issues directly, but might find it safer to present dreams that reveal their concerns in a metaphorical manner.

Dreams prior to termination can be indicators of how clients feel about the end of treatment (Cavenar & Nash, 1976). Clients may be trying to communicate indirectly with therapists through such dreams about their readiness or lack of readiness to terminate from treatment. For example, depending on the personal associations, a dream that a client was graduating from college with high honors might indicate readiness to terminate, whereas a dream that a client was drowning or murdered might indicate lack of readiness to terminate.

In addition, changes in dream images over the course of therapy can indicate changes in the person's level of functioning (see review of research in Chapter 12). For example, one client began therapy with a recurrent dream about waves washing over her. By the end of therapy, she no longer had the recurrent dream but had dreams where she was in a peaceful setting with other people. The changes in the dream content reflected the symptomalogical and interpersonal changes she had made in therapy. In contrast, repetition of a recurrent dream about being murdered might be an indication that the person is not changing and that either a different strategy or a referral is needed.

USING DREAM IMAGES AS METAPHORS IN THERAPY

Once some understanding of the images in dreams has been reached, therapists can use these images as metaphors to bridge back into talking about other therapeutic issues. Incorporating images from dreams as metaphors in subsequent therapy can provide a continuity between dream interpretation and other therapeutic techniques. Using dream images can help to form a powerful bond of communication similar to the use of metaphors in therapy (Hill & Regan, 1991). Metaphors seem particularly useful because they tap into our nonverbal imaging and intuitive experiencing and give a person a picture to hang on to that symbolizes the issue.

As an example, one client presented a dream in which she was swimming blindfolded; the interpretation revealed that she was avoiding a major issue in her life. We later used the dream image of swimming blindfolded to refer to her avoidance of things that she did not want to cope with. The phrase "swimming blindfolded" was a metaphor for her problem with avoidance.

Another client reported a dream in which she was trapped in a cage in a jungle. We used this image as a metaphor throughout the remainder of brief therapy to talk about how she felt trapped. As we talked about it more, she came to realize that the cage both imprisoned her but also protected her from the dangers of the jungle. She decided that she would like to keep the cage so that she could go in when she wanted protection but have it unlocked so that she could get out when she wanted.

THE IMPORTANCE OF THE THERAPEUTIC RELATIONSHIP

Many theorists have discussed the importance of the therapeutic relationship in psychotherapy (e.g., Bordin, 1979; Gelso & Carter, 1985, 1994; Rogers, 1957), with some focusing particularly on the relationship in dream interpretation (Bonime, 1987; Ullman, 1987). Furthermore, a great deal of research has shown that the working alliance is one of the best predictors of therapeutic outcome (Horvath & Symonds, 1991; Orlinsky, Grawe, & Parks, 1994). Interestingly, however, the evidence shows that it is the client's perception of the alliance rather than the therapist's perception that makes the most difference in terms of client outcome (Gurman, 1977; Horvath, 1995). Thus, it is not so important that the therapist believes that he or she is understanding but that the client perceives the therapist as being understanding. Therapists have often mistakenly believed that they had a good therapeutic relationship when in fact clients have not revealed their dissatisfactions, believing that therapists did not want to hear or feeling that they did not want to confront or upset the therapist (Hill et al., 1993).

Different kinds of alliances might be necessary with different clients. For example, some clients want a very empathic therapist who understands their feelings and communicates support. Other clients are threatened by too much support and want the therapist to be more distant and withholding. It is the therapist's job to figure out how to relate to different clients rather than assuming that clients should adjust to his or her style.

A sense of collaboration between the therapist and client is essential. In fact, one could argue that a good relationship is particularly crucial for dream interpretation because clients make themselves so vulnerable, opening up areas of themselves when they are not sure what is going to be revealed.

The therapist is not the expert who provides the client with "the" interpretation of his or her dream. Rather, therapists serve as facilitators in this model to help clients explore their dreams, always respecting the privacy of the dreamer. In this model, therapists serve as collaborators in constructing the meaning of the dreams with the clients. Therapists also work with clients by prompting associations, reflecting feelings, offering tentative interpretations, challenging defenses, and suggesting possible action plans, but the client always has the final say about what fits. Therapists must respect clients and appreciate that clients need to have a sense of responsibility for, or "owning" of, the interpretation or action.

I agree with Ullman (1979, 1987; Ullman & Zimmerman, 1979) that the dreamer has the exclusive authority about the meaning of the dream. The therapist's job is to stimulate the dreamer to think about the meaning of the dream rather than to impose meaning from outside. Given that the dream is stimulated by the dreamer's thoughts, no one else can ever really know what these thoughts mean to him or her. Hence, we need to respect that the dreamer has the key to the dream and work with the dreamer to facilitate his or her exploration of the dream.

MONITORING CLIENT RESPONSIVENESS TO DREAM INTERPRETATION

Throughout dream interpretation, as with all of therapy, therapists need to remember to pay attention to the interaction. Therapists need to be aware of how clients are responding to each stage. They need to determine if clients value dream interpretation and want to participate in it. They need to ask clients how they feel about doing dream interpretation. Rather than forcing dream interpretation on clients, therapists need to assess continually how clients are responding. We know that clients often do not tell us when they feel negatively about certain therapist interventions (Hill, Thompson, & Corbett, 1992; Hill, Thompson et al., 1993; Regan & Hill, 1992; Thompson & Hill, 1991), so we cannot assume that clients are as enthusiastic about dream interpretation as we might be. Kiesler's (1988) theory about meta-communication is of great utility here in providing guidance for therapists about how to discuss what is going on in the interaction with the client. He suggested that at moments when clients appear to be upset, therapists state what they personally are feeling and ask clients how they are feeling, prompting a discussion of the relationship. By talking about the relationship, clients can often be helped to communicate more effectively and learn that it is permissible to discuss their feelings openly in therapy.

Therapists also need to monitor whether clients can handle the intensity of reexperiencing feelings and the depth of self-examination that dream interpretation requires. Dream interpretation can be threatening for some clients. I recommend that therapists progress slowly during an initial dream interpretation and determine how the client is responding at each step. Therapists might want to steer clients away from the intense feelings brought up by their dreams if clients get frightened by the affect in the dream or begin to dissociate. Rather than going intensely into the feelings associated with the images in the dream with such clients, therapists might want either to stick to a more cognitive interpretation or to wait until later in the therapy to do dream interpretation when the client can handle the intensity that dream interpretation can require.

On the other hand, some clients are resistant to getting into feelings and need to be confronted to go deeper. Dream content often suggests areas that people are avoiding. For example, if a person says that everything in his life is fine, but his dreams are filled with violence and destruction, the therapist has a clue that should be followed up. Obviously, clinical experience is needed to determine when to back off and when to confront.

THE NEED FOR FLEXIBILITY

I recommend that beginning therapists follow the model fairly closely the first few times they use it. After using it a few times, therapists can use this model as a framework within which to work and can modify it to fit their style and the needs of clients.

Rather than sticking rigidly to exactly the way that I have presented the model, I am more concerned that therapists learn the theory behind this method of dream interpretation. With a thorough understanding of the theory, therapists can pick and choose the specific techniques than will help them attain their goals. The theory (as explicated in Chapters 4 through 7) is that dreams reflect the individual's waking life and so the dreamer needs to explore personal associations in an emotionally arousing manner to lead to insight, changes in cognitive schemata, and changed behaviors. Therapists need to think about what their goals are within each of the three stages and try to determine how best to help their clients attain the goals.

I would caution, however, that therapists should be especially careful not to cut the Exploration Stage short. Without the strong foundation of an exploration of the feelings and cognitions of the dreamer, a therapist cannot come up with a helpful interpretation of the meaning of a specific dream even when he or she has extensive knowledge of a dreamer. In addition, however, I would note that therapists need to leave enough time for the Insight and Action Stages; some therapists get so caught up in exploring every single image that they have no time left for putting the dream all together and determining a course of action.

A complete dream interpretation using this method usually takes at least a full therapy hour and often two to three sessions. Therapists should not rush through the stages because the in-depth processing of the material seems to be what makes a difference in helping clients understand the richness and complexity of their personal associations to dream images. Often there is some blurring of stages, with therapists jumping to do interpretations or returning to do more associations during the Insight and Action Stages. Such blurring is fine as long as therapists complete all three stages.

COUNTERTRANSFERENCE ISSUES

As with any emotionally evocative topic in therapy, interpreting dreams has the potential for stimulating countertransference feelings (a loss of objectivity based on strong internal reactions to the client). Primitive emotions or behaviors that are expressed in dreams may be disconcerting or repugnant to therapists, causing them to veer away from exploring these parts of dreams. Or therapists might have such strong associations or interpretations based on their own issues that it is hard for them to hear clients' associations or interpretations. Therapists need to think carefully through these issues so that they can understand them and try not to let them adversely influence the therapy that they offer.

Therapists' dreams about clients might reflect countertransference issues. Although therapists probably will not choose to talk about these issues with clients in therapy, an awareness of such dreams can help them clarify the issues in their own minds. For example, a dream about having a romantic interlude with a client might suggest that the therapist has strong sexual attraction to the client and needs to monitor his or her behavior in therapy. Or it might suggest that the client has been seductive in therapy and the therapist has not been aware of it consciously but has been reacting to it at another level. One therapist had a dream that she was trying to clean her client's house but that she was getting angry because the client's spouse kept getting in her way. This dream alerted the therapist that her feelings of anger toward the spouse were interfering with her focusing on the client's responsibility in this situation.

A strong pull in dream interpretation seems to be the desire of therapists to tell clients what their dreams mean. Perhaps therapists feel a need to show off their brilliance or intuitiveness at being able to make sense of the dream and connect it to underlying client dynamics. Or perhaps therapists get pulled into clients' desires to have someone tell them the meaning of dreams that seem external to them. Or perhaps therapists get impatient going through the long and sometimes tedious process of carefully mining the associations and helping the clients come to their own understandings. In this model, therapists serve as coaches and guides, which can be frustrating and ungratifying for some therapists. Therapists obviously need to choose the approach that fit with their needs and styles, but also need to be aware when their own issues interfere with client growth.

One way for therapists to assess whether countertransference is occurring is to examine how far they have strayed from the model. Perhaps a therapist fails to ask for associations to certain images, fails to reflect particular feelings implied in some of the associations, pushes a specific interpretation, fails to notice when the client becomes quiet and the therapist is doing all the work, or skips the Action Stage. These deviations could be evidence that the client is not ready or able to handle a particular emotion or interpretation, but the deviation could also reflect countertransference due to the therapist's feeling threatened personally by the dream material. Dreams are particularly evocative and easily tap into unresolved material for therapists.

In situations when countertransference becomes a problem, I recommend that therapists seek consultation and supervision. I view supervision as an necessity for therapists throughout the span of their careers because doing therapy has a way of constantly stimulating personal issues. I doubt that dream interpretation stimulates more countertransference issues than other types of interventions but would stress that therapists always need to be vigilant to ensure that they are providing the best services possible for their clients.

SUMMARY

There are a number of clinical issues to think about when applying this model. Therapists will probably use dream interpretation mostly with clients who have positive attitudes about dreams, who are motivated to understand their dreams, and/or who have troubling dreams. Therapists need to establish a good therapeutic relationship with clients. They also need to monitor client responsiveness to dream interpretation, not interpreting dreams if clients either do not have dreams or do not want to talk about their dreams, or if dream interpretation causes clients to become frightened because of the intensity of the feelings that sometimes get aroused. Flexibility in using the model is suggested, with therapists being urged to think about the theory underlying the model (that dreams reflect waking life so the goal of dream interpretation is to get the dreamer to explore personal associations in an emotionally arousing manner to lead to insight, changes in schemata, and changed behaviors). Specific suggestions are given for introducing the importance of dreams early in therapy; for asking about dreams at times of impasse, intense transference, or termination; for using dream images as metaphors later in therapy as a follow-up to dream interpretation; and for managing countertransference feelings.

PART III

❧

Clinical Examples of Using the Cognitive–Experiential Model in Therapy

Single-Session
Dream Interpretation

THE FOLLOWING EXCERPT is presented as an illustration of working with dreams with a client in a single session. Although dream interpretation is usually done within the context of ongoing psychotherapy, this session shows that therapists can also work with dreams just in a single session, particularly with highly functioning people. I chose this example because it provides a good demonstration of all the stages of the model and because it shows how much background information therapists can learn about clients through working with a dream. Therapists do not have to have lots of history prior to the dream interpretation because much of the relevant material will emerge through talking about the images in the dream.

The client was an attractive, perky, female 20-year-old undergraduate college student majoring in psychology who volunteered to participate in a study on dream interpretation. I was the therapist (at the time I was a 46-year-old professor of counseling psychology). The client read the transcript of this session and gave her written consent for it to be used in this book.

The transcript has been edited to make it shorter and easier to read, but the content of the dialogue has not been altered. The beginnings of the three stages are indicated so that readers can refer back to the dream interpretation model. C stands for client and T stands for therapist in the transcript.

EXPLORATION STAGE

T: So what I want to do is have you tell me your dream. If you can, tell it to me as if you are experiencing it right now. Then we're going to go through and look at what the dream means to you.

The Dream

1 remember standing out at our shore house. It was probably like in early evening, not too late because the sun was setting. I just remember, this sounds so crazy, these two huge sharks. This guy was standing there with me. I have no idea who he was; he didn't really have a face. He wasn't anyone that I knew. He fell in and was eaten by a shark. Then later my boyfriend, we have a puppy together (laugh) *came out. I was like, "Don't go near the water," but our puppy went near the water. He was still little and always gets into everything. He was looking in the water. He didn't fall into the water because I grabbed him by the collar. So I saved our puppy* (laugh).

T: What I'm going to do is ask you to associate to the different parts of the dream. When I say associate, I mean tell me anything that comes to mind when you think of that thing.

C: Okay.

T: So tell me about the shore house.

C: My grandparents have had the shore house all of my life. I've spent every summer down there. So, just a lot of really good memories, like going fishing with my grandfather, just a big family time. So, how I feel about that is, part of it is really good. But these past two summers have been really different for me. I'm a junior in college. I spend a month at my home in Pennsylvania, and then I live 9 months here, and then I go to the shore for the summer. And it's like, *(laugh)* where's my house? That's been like a hard thing because I have such close ties with my family, like everybody knows everything about everybody's life, and it's great. And I think I'm having a hard time dealing with the separation, like, you know, time to grow up. I like the independence, but at the same time, like last night I was so upset and stressed. I just want my mom *(laugh)*. I'm sure that's how most college students are. But it's been good because going from such an independent atmosphere at college and then going back to your home and having all the rules and "be in at this time" . . . whatever, has been kind of difficult. At the shore my grandparents would be down every weekend, but during the week my two brothers and I had the house to ourselves. It was neat, but at the same time it was kind of like should I be doing this now or should I be waiting until I really have to be on my own. You know what I mean?

T: I'm not quite sure. Go back to that part for me.

C: I mean I'm 20 years old, at the time that I should get a little more independent. I do a lot of things on my own, and I take care of things that I never would have, like finances. Like in high school I never worried about that. So now I'm beginning to realize what the real world is like. But after spending 9 months at school and having all that independence, it's kind of nice to go back home and not worry about it. You know what I mean?

T: So you would have liked to have been with the family?

C: Probably, I mean, I think so, but then when I'm with them, I just want to go back to school, so it's kind of like a "catch-22."

T: So it's a transition time, figuring out who you are and where you're going.

C: Right.

T: Next you were on the dock.

C: Yeah, the dock is so pretty. We have a big bay window and we always eat dinner as a family together there. It's so relaxing on the bay. People think it's so weird that I'd rather be on the bay side than on the beach front, but there's fishing there and the sailboats. I always go swimming off the dock, and I love fishing (*laugh*).

T: So it sounds like it's really the spot where everything happens.

C: Right. It's where all the action is.

T: Sharks.

C: Sharks. Let's see. I love shark fishing. That's something my older brother and I do. I'm not 21, so I don't go to the bars. I don't really drink anyway. We'd be sitting there and wouldn't know what to do. None of us had to work late at night, so we would go shark fishing (*laugh*). So I don't really know about sharks. I like sharks, I think they're cool. But the stereotype around sharks is they're evil and stuff like that.

T: So there's two parts of it. Sharks are cool. They're kind of neat animals. But there's danger associated with sharks.

C: Right. Yeah. That's how I see it.

T: Why are they cool?

C: I don't know. I think they're just like really neat. I love the ocean. The only thing I really hate are jellyfish. Sharks don't bother me at all (*laugh*). I don't know why. I used to be terrified of the water when I was little, and I would never go into the ocean because I was like, "A shark's gonna get me." But it's not because I ever saw the movie "Jaws." It's just something you always hear as a child, "Sharks are bad." My dad was a lifeguard for 12 years, and he said, "You don't ever have to worry about sharks getting you; you're more likely to be hit by lightning." So once he put it in that perspective for me, then I was like, "It's not a big deal, they're not going to attack me."

T: So you got over your fear through his reassurance.

C: Yeah, I got over my fear really easily and then I spent every second in the water (*laugh*) down at the shore. I just think those animals are kind of cool (*laugh*).

T: What do they epitomize to you?

C: I don't know. I just think it's neat to be in the water. I like swimming. I used to swim in high school and I'm a swim coach now (*laugh*). I just think the water is a really neat thing to me. In fact, I remember having dreams where I thought it would be cool if our whole house was filled with water and you could swim around. I have very few dreams that recur, but that is one of them. So the water for me has always symbolized something really neat, really exciting, like you can explore and stuff like that. So I think sharks are a neat thing because they are associated with water.

T: You kind of identify with them in some way.

C: Right, right.

T: What do you like about sharks that you don't like about other fish though? How are they different?

C: (*laugh*) They have more personality. It sounds strange, but like, a flounder's just a flounder—it's ugly. It has eyes on one side of its head. We like going shark fishing on the dock. You put a big spotlight there and wait for the small fish and the sharks come eventually. I just remember sitting there watching my uncles shark fishing when I was little. I always thought it would be so much fun (*laugh*).

T: Because they're big and powerful and . . . ?

C: Yeah, and just the way they move through the water.

T: They're kind of sensuous?

C: Yeah, they curve around, which is neat. Other fish are just there, they all look the same.

T: There's nothing real distinctive.

C: Yeah. Exactly.

T: The shark is the top of the pack . . .

C: (*laugh*) Oh yeah . . .

T: And these were huge sharks.

C: Yeah. In my dream they were really big. Usually in our bay we've caught small sharks, but these sharks were huge.

T: So kind of like the lion is the king of the jungle, and the shark is king of the ocean, king of the bay.

C: Right, yeah (*laugh*).

T: There were two of them.

C: Yeah. I don't know why actually. The only thing I can think of is that I have this thing with even numbers. My favorite number is 24. I set my alarm clock for, like 8:04, never 8:03. It can't be an odd number or my day is going to be bad.

T: There was a guy standing next to you who didn't have a face. You didn't know who he was.

C: Right. I don't know how I knew he was a guy. He just was a guy. He was bigger than me, but he wasn't threatening to me at all. I just remember him standing there hanging out at the dock looking at the sharks and then all of a sudden he fell in. He didn't have a face, and he wasn't anyone I knew.

T: He didn't have a face, or you couldn't see his face?

C: I couldn't see his face. When I dream, like I don't see people. It's more of a feeling. Like I knew that was my boyfriend, and I knew that was our dog. So it's not like anyone really has a face. It was just more like he was just an unknown to me.

T: Uh huh. Anything about him that . . .

C: There was nothing about him really in particular. He was just there, and he didn't say anything to me or do anything. He just fell in the water (*laugh*) and was eaten by a shark (*laugh*).

T: So compared to the shark, he didn't have any personality.

C: Right (*laugh*), exactly (*laugh*).

T: Falling into water. What does that . . . ?

C: (*pause*) I don't know. I don't have a fear of water. I don't know if it would mean anything. Recently I've been so stressed out. Usually I handle things really well, but this semester has just been totally overwhelming. So I don't know if falling in would have anything, like falling in, you're trapped, you don't know what you're going to do. Like last night I was so upset for no reason. I had a great night, I had coached for two hours, I had a great time. Then I got back to my boyfriend's house, and I was studying for my exam. I wasn't that stressed out about my exam, but I just lost it and started to cry. I usually never cry, like nothing really ever upsets me. And he's like, "What's wrong?" And I was like, "I don't know, I just want to go home (*laugh*) and see my mom and dad." It was just really weird. And this morning when I woke up, I was just like, I don't know what that was all about. It was just not characteristic of me at all.

T: So something's going on in your life.

C: Yeah, I would think so, but I really don't know what it is, and that's bothering me.

T: Well, it sure sounds like there is some danger. Those sharks are circling around. If you fall in, the sharks can get you.

C: Right. Yeah. But I wasn't worried about me falling in. I was more worried about . . .

T: . . . Taking care of everybody else.

C: Yeah.

T: I mean this guy next to you falls in.

C: Right.

T: But you didn't try to save him in the dream.

C: No, I didn't try to save him. I don't know if that was because I didn't see it when it happened or if I didn't know him. I didn't react as quickly as I usually would.

T: Uh huh. You didn't seem to do anything much at that point.

C: Right. I was just standing there and realized he fell in (*laugh*) and that was basically it.

T: Uh huh. Tell me about your boyfriend.

C: We've been together almost 2 years. He's wonderful, I love him to death, and eventually we plan to get married. I mean, I'm still young and I know that. We met my freshman year. The last thing I wanted was a boyfriend, and the last thing he wanted was a girlfriend. We just met each other, and it was like magic. He is so awesome. He's really different from any guy that I've ever met. He's really sensitive. He tells me how he feels all the time. It's so nice, because I like to be reassured a lot, I think because my dad was always like that. It's like I'm Daddy's girl. He's a lot like my father. He's a lot like my younger brother too, because my younger brother wants everything to be perfect and anytime something is wrong in the family, he's always the one trying to work it out.

T: So your boyfriend's like that too.

C: Yeah. My boyfriend's like that too. He's like a lot of the men in my family. I respect my grandfather tremendously, and my father, and my older brother is my best friend in the whole world. And I see a lot of similarities with my brother. I think that's what I like about him. Like even some things that I hate about my older brother, I see in my boyfriend. I just like it because it's something familiar to me. Yet he's really different from them also, which is really nice. I mean I can't really say anything bad about him.

T: You said he reminds you so much of the other men in your family, so there's some kind of connection there with family.

C: Right, yeah. He's met my brother. My brother has never liked any guy that I've ever dated, but when he met my boyfriend, he was like, "This guy's great," which is good because I knew I was right. I really have a lot of faith in my brother's judgment. My dad likes him. It's really important that my family likes him because I'm so close to my family, and I wouldn't want to be with anyone that would cause problems with that.

T: Yeah. It sounds like your family is just very special.

C: Yeah, I think so. It's really neat the way that my family is. A lot of my friends always wanted to be with my family.

T: Tell me about the puppy.

C: We just got him. I love puppies. The puppy is a black Lab. My boyfriend loves dogs, so I wanted to get him this puppy. He's such a good puppy. We have a good time with him. Our friends are like, "Oh, he's like your child, that's so sick" (*laugh*). Thank god, it's not a child. I would not want a kid (*laugh*) after taking care of the puppy—such a huge responsibility. But we don't regret it. My parents think I'm nuts (*laugh*).

T: Why?

C: They're like, "You have enough to worry about." But it's something that I need. Like I go and take the puppy for a walk. We'll go down to the park, and I'll play with him for an hour. And, like, it's a time where I don't have to think about anything besides having fun, and for me it's good. And the same with coaching swimming. I coach 7-, 8-, and 9-year-olds, and I just totally concentrate on them, which is good because it gets kind of overwhelming sometimes. But it's the same with the puppy as it is with coaching. It's just like a release to do something else.

T: Uh huh. So, lots of responsibility but lots of fun, like a baby.

C: Yeah.

T: It's interesting because when you first said it, you said you and your boyfriend had a puppy together, kind of like having a baby together.

C: I know. He's our joint responsibility, like when we take him to the vet everything is 50/50, just because he's expensive. My mentality about that is, like, I can spend money on a puppy or I can spend money on going out and drinking, like most college students. I don't do that, so I can afford a dog.

T: Just given the way you said it, you and your boyfriend having the puppy together, did getting it mean a greater commitment in your relationship?

C: I don't, see, that's interesting. I don't, I think sort of. It's kind of like, we feel this way. If something changes, then it'll change. But as of now, we feel like we're the right ones for each other. But, yeah I mean, this is *our* dog. Like we don't really own anything together, but he's ours. And yeah, I think it symbolizes like a greater commitment. Nothing like serious, but he's our little puppy (*laugh*), and that's kind of neat. I didn't really think about it at the time, but I definitely see that.

T: You used the contrast that other students don't have dogs. So this gives you something more permanent.

C: Right, yeah. There are, like a friend of mine has a dog. I feel really bad for some college dogs because college students aren't really that responsible (*laugh*). Like I see them giving beer to the dog and that really bothers me. No one is ever going to give our dog any beer because I think that is horrible. I'm like so protective over him.

T: In the dream, the puppy went to the water, and you warned your boyfriend and the dog not to go to the water. The dog went to the water and fell in, and you were very worried in the dream about protecting your dog.

C: Yeah (*laugh*), I don't know. For me this dream is really bizarre. It just is funny.

T: It sounds like it's a little embarrassing.

C: Yeah. I've always thought dreams are really neat, and when I dream, I wonder what it means. It's something that I've always been really interested in, but I think that's why I think it's so funny that I have this dream.

T: Yeah, I'm struck by the fact that there are a lot of different messages, with the dog particularly.

C: Right.

T: But the guy drowns. I mean you let him. But you're very, very concerned about and very protective of the dog and your boyfriend, but it feels funny and you have some embarrassment around that.

C: Yeah, because it sounds so crazy.

T: But you don't feel as embarrassed at all by letting this other guy drown.

C: Somebody can be drowning and I don't even think twice about it. God forbid my dog drowns (*laugh*). But, I'm very protective over anyone in my family or anyone I care about. It's been bad in some senses because, like my older brother . . . I remember I was up visiting him my senior year in high school for siblings weekend. We went to a party and he got into a fight, and I jumped in and punched this guy in the mouth and I knocked his tooth out (*laugh*). It was awful because I didn't even think twice about it. It was just something that was done. I mean his fraternity brothers, thank God, were there because I don't know what the guy would have done because he was totally shocked that I did that. But that's something that I've done. When I was younger, I was a tomboy and we would always do stuff together. We would always play together. But I'd be right there too in the fights. That's why I tell my boyfriend not to ever get in a fight. If you're gonna do it, make sure I am nowhere around, because . . .

T: Don't ever get into the water.

C: Don't ever get near the water (*laugh*), because I'll jump in. And he's like, "Why would you do that, that's stupid." And I was like, "I know, now that I think about it, I know it's stupid." But I can't even, like . . .

T: Your boyfriend didn't go near the water.

C: No, he didn't go near the water. He listened to me (*laugh*).

T: Is that true in life? Would he be pretty cautious?

C: Yeah. He really cares a lot about how I feel and what I think. He asks me for advice a lot. I'm the same way with him, like we communicate really well. We're really open with each other, and we don't fight often. When we do, it's just because someone's not listening to someone else. Like with studying, I study a lot. I prepare myself, and I do well in school. And he does well, but he doesn't do as well as me GPA-wise. But I'm in psychology, and he's in chemistry and physics—I would drown in those classes. So he sees like last semester I got a 4.0 and he got a 3.4, which is great, but he's like, "What are you doing that I'm not doing?" The way that I study—I take notes on yellow pads and then rewrite them, and I read all my chapters before class so it's more familiar to me because a lot of teachers pull things right from the book, and I type out review sheets. He has started to do a lot of things that I've done, and that's really good for him. And for me, like I would spend so much time studying that I would never go out and have a good time. When I met him, he was totally like the opposite. He was going out all the time. He was on the swim team, and they would go out every night drinking like crazy. I met him when he was swimming, so he wasn't drinking. He was being really good. Thank God I met him then because (*laugh*) I never would have met him otherwise. So we've come to find a common ground. He's helped me relax a little bit more, and I've helped him become more serious.

T: So you used to be more worried about taking care of him.

C: Yeah. He slips sometimes and calls me "Mom." I talk to his parents a lot. I'm really close to them too. It's funny because his mom and I think a lot alike. I get really goofy and do crazy things and I'm not even drunk (*laugh*). He just thinks it's so funny because his mom is the same way. She's just crazy. She dances around at restaurants. She always lives for the day and has a good time. His dad is a lot like my boyfriend. He's more like, "What's up, dude?" I laugh at him, so it's kind of neat. We're more like his parents than we are like mine, which is fine.

T: How are your parents?

C: My parents don't drink. My mom was married when she was 19. My dad was 20. She went to college for a semester and then met my dad. My dad actually was friends with my mom's parents first. He waited until she went to college and asked her parents if it was okay for him to ask my mom for a date. They started dating and got married and had four kids. It's great because my mom has always wanted that, and she's a wonderful mother. She would always go to my games. My father was the same way. He worked, but he went out on disability the end of my junior year. He was there all the time. Just they're more centered on family than my boyfriend's parents where it's just the four of them really who are close. My parents don't go out a lot. My dad always wants to do more than my mom does. My mom is happiest in her home. I don't know if that's because she's insecure being outside the family because that's really all she knows. Like, I look at my life—I'm 20 years old, and I've experienced a lot more and know a lot more than she did when she was 20. I mean, she was married when she was 19 and pregnant when she was 20. But they're just different, I mean, I love them, they're great parents, but like my mom and I are really different.

T: So . . . let me just get back. You were saying that you and your boyfriend are more like his parents.

C: Yeah.

T: Your parents are a little bit more stable.

C: Yeah. They're definitely more stable. They are really involved in the community and school. She's so good at stuff like this, and I really respect my mom for that a lot. I respect my dad a lot too, but in different ways. But I see my mom as being different than me. Like I want a career, I want to go to graduate school and get my doctorate in psychology. It's just something that she was never really geared to do. Sometimes that causes problems. Like last year I got a 3.8 and a 4.0, and I was so excited. My dad could totally understand. He was like, "That's great." And my mom, like, she did say like, "Good job," but I wanted her to get a little more excited. But she doesn't really know what that's like. I also see that she didn't want to make a big deal out of my grade point average because of my older brother and my older sister, like she doesn't want them to feel bad.

T: She's always protecting them, kind of like you are.

C: Right, we've talked about this a lot lately. Like we used to not get along at all. We used to always be at each other's throat. Now I understand her more, and I was like, "We're just different, that's good because I can learn a lot from you and you can learn a lot from me. We just have to look at it like that and not have you try to change me to be this way and not have me try to change you." Since we've had our little talk, everything's been fine. I felt she wanted me to be more like her, but I could always relate more to my brother and my father because I played soccer with my brother all through childhood. My dad was our coach. My mom wasn't in sports. I think that was hard for her because I'm supposed to be a little girl. I'm supposed to fit these neat little generalizations, and I didn't really quite go with that.

INSIGHT STAGE

T: Let's try to put together what you've said so far and try to figure out what this dream is about. What do you think it means?

C: I think a lot of it is about the separation. It's time to move on to my own things. I'm beginning to look at grad schools. I might go far away from my family, which for me is kind of hard, but it's kind of exciting at the same time. I don't want to leave them because I know they'll miss me, and I know my mom worries about me all the time. She's written me three letters in one week, and I know she's worried about me right now.

T: You mentioned a couple of times that you're feeling overwhelmed, a lot of stress now. What's going on that's particularly difficult right now?

C: I think I'm not doing as well in school as I think I should be doing. I have Bs but it's kind of frustrating. And I haven't been home in a while. I haven't seen my sister in a long time. My phone bills are awful (*laugh*). So I don't know. I'm just feeling overwhelmed. It's hard to study at my house. My roommates go out a lot and play loud music when they're getting ready to go out. So I study over at my boyfriend's house, which works fine for me, but I kind of get aggravated with them because I should be able to study at my house. And they're so messy, and that's really annoying (*laugh*). I don't know what else is really stressful.

T: The sharks seem more dangerous. If you think of sharks circling, you know, they eat this guy. I mean that's dangerous.

C: That is pretty dangerous.

T: And your puppy is in danger.

C: Yeah.

T: So, it sounds like somehow someone is in danger.

C: Yeah. The only thing I can think of is, like I definitely had a good summer. I met a lot of nice people. But at the same time I don't want to spend another summer there. I feel like I need something else. I worked on the beach as a beach checker . . . checked tags. It's a really hard job. I knew, like, all the lifeguards, who were mostly guys. My boyfriend was kind of nervous about that. My brother did not like these two guards that I was really good friends with, probably because he liked my boyfriend so much. That was hard for me because I've always gotten, like, along with my brother really, really well. And like we didn't even talk for the longest time. I would just try to avoid him. It wasn't like the summer before when we'd talk about serious things like his girlfriend and my boyfriend.

T: There was a lot of tension.

C: Yeah, there was a little tension. And then there was a fraternity fire. On the news they were just saying a fraternity. We weren't sure which one burned down. There were six people dead, and my mom was in hysterics. So I was like great, that's the last thing I need. Not getting along with my brother and then God forbid something happens to him.

T: When did this happen?

C: This was really recently. This was not even a week ago. It just happened.

T: Was it around the time of the dream?

C: Yeah, actually, that was probably around the same time.

T: That makes some sense, doesn't it?

C: Yeah, it definitely makes some sense. Then my brother called my mom and said he was fine. It wasn't his fraternity. But my brother was good friends with two of the guys that died, and my mom was really worried about my brother. She's like, "Maybe you want to call and see what's going on." Because my parents know that I'm really close to my brother and like if he's going to tell anyone anything, he'll tell me. I'm really worried about him too. Last spring one of his fraternity brothers drank himself to death, and my brother was the one who gave him CPR and tried to bring him back. He never really said anything about that, just "I'm fine, I'm fine." That's all he would say. And then now two of his other friends, like I don't know, I think that'd be really hard.

T: So there is some pretty good danger.

C: Yeah. And he's not saying anything about it. If that happened to me, I'd need to talk to someone. I don't know if it's better for him, but I don't see it as being really good, because he's not really telling anyone anything, not even his girlfriend. It's always like he's fine, plays the macho role, "I'm not too worried about it." And like when I call, he's like, "I really don't have anything to say, I've dealt with things, everything's fine."

T: You seem to be worried about him.

C: Yeah, I don't know how to get through to him. If he doesn't want to talk to you, then he doesn't, he just keeps pushing you away. I guess that could be part of the danger (*laugh*). So, I don't know, that's all I can think of.

T: Well, it sounds like it hits a pretty good core there.

C: Yeah, it does (*laugh*). I didn't really think of that.

T: You did start out saying that things were tense at the beach this summer.

C: Yeah, things were tense. And I think once I see him again, I hope he'll be able to say something to me about how he's feeling because I think then I'll feel better. But until then, I think that's something I'm worrying about.

T: It's kind of interesting. I keep coming back to this image of this one guy going in the water and getting eaten up, which shows how much danger is there. You weren't concerned with him, but then the puppy, somebody that is close to you, was real, and you had to protect your puppy.

C: Is that why I did that (*laugh*)? I've always been like I'm always worried about people that I'm close to, and I always want everything to be Okay with them, and I totally go out of my way to do stuff for people.

T: Who does your puppy remind you of in your life?

C: My puppy? I don't know.

T: You described "our" puppy in terms of someone that you have to take responsibility for and take care of so much.

C: My brother (*laugh*).

T: That's a pretty good parallel.

C: Yeah, that's kind of weird. He's my older brother, but he kind of shuts himself off from my parents. Like we all get along, but he feels like he's the black sheep of the family. He's made mistakes in his life, so have I, but being the oldest son, he's supposed to be perfect. He's the one who is gifted. He doesn't think he has to work, whereas I've internalized the belief that I'm average, so I feel that I have to work harder, and I do, so I do better, but he doesn't understand that. He thinks that things come easy to me. He thinks that my parents pay for all of my college, which is extremely untrue. I'm the third kid in college. My dad is disabled and in the middle of a lawsuit. I have a lot of loans, which is fine, I'll pay them off, I'm not really worried about that. But he has a misconception that my parents take care of me first and then him, because he has loans too, and he gets kind of angry about things.

T: This explains some of the [tension] between the two of you.

C: Yeah, definitely, because I am Daddy's girl. My dad is the disciplinarian in our family and I can get away with stuff. I don't get upset often, but when I do, like, I let people know. I'll curse in front of my parents. I won't curse at them, but I'll curse about something I'm upset about in general. And they won't say anything, they'll let me go. But if my brother starts cursing, they'll make him knock it off. But if anything goes wrong with my older brother, I'll feel guilty, like I could have done something. Because it's always like my mom asks me to call him and see what's wrong because they're at a loss, they don't know what else to do.

T: So the responsibility is coming from your parents.

C: Right, right.

T: And he doesn't want to talk to you.

C: No, he doesn't want to talk to me because he knows he's in the wrong with things. I told him, "You shouldn't be drinking as much as you are." Alcoholism runs in our family, that's something that I get nervous about, and my parents get nervous about. My dad's not an alcoholic, but he just doesn't drink with his blood pressure medicine. My mom said that before they got married, he was out drinking with her father and when he came back he was obnoxious, so she told him, "You're annoying when you drink." So he just said, "I don't want to be annoying." So I think that's another reason why he doesn't. But I just see my brother as floating along and not knowing where to ground himself. That makes me nervous.

T: It's interesting. With a puppy you have a lot more control.

C: Yeah (*laugh*), yeah, I do.

T: It sounds like the frustrating part with him is he won't talk to you. He's figured out how to shut you out.

C: Yeah.

T: It's almost more like that guy without the face in a way. It's hard to get a connection with him.

C: Right.

T: I wonder if that's the fear. You'd like him to be a puppy that you could rescue, but the fear is that he's the guy that just is going to get swallowed up and eaten by a shark.

C: That's really good. Yeah, because I was totally in control, like I just grabbed the dog's collar, and he was fine.

T: And your brother hasn't got a collar that you can grab.

C: Right, exactly, this other person just died.

T: It was out of your control. There was nothing you could do.

C: That's cool. I didn't think of that. I wouldn't have even thought about where to start with that at all.

T: Well, it's frustrating because you care for him a lot.

C: Yeah, I'm sure it'll work out, but at this point it's just frustrating and stressful because it's always something in the back of my mind that I worry about. I don't bring it up to the surface because there's nothing I can do.

T: I was just thinking about his drinking. I was thinking of the metaphor of drinking like a fish.

C: Yeah (*laugh*), that's my brother (*laugh*). Yeah, that's true.

ACTION STAGE

T: The next step is to try to figure out what you want to do.

C: How about put a collar on him (*laugh*)?

T: It would be nice if you could do that.

C: Yeah, right.

T: But then again you talked about how much responsibility a dog is, and I don't think you want more responsibility.

C: Really, I talked to my mom about my brother. He's almost out of college. He's out of our hands, I mean out of *my parents'* hands. Oh my God, that's awful. He's out of *their* control.

T: He's not your responsibility.

C: Yeah, that's really hard for me. That's just the way I am. Like, I mean, it's stressful, but I couldn't just say I'm not going to talk to him, I'm not going to deal with it, because for me that would be even worse.

T: That would feel too terrible, just to stand there and let him drown.

C: Yeah, right. But there's only so much you can do. I told my parents, "You just let him know that you know he's got to work things out on his own. So if he doesn't want to do well in school, then he's gonna pay the price." I said, "Let him know that you love him. That's all you can do because you can't always pick up the pieces. He's got to learn for himself." Like he borrows money like crazy. He's so irresponsible. He made so much money this summer, and he spent two months of this money on a friendship ring for his girlfriend. That would be nice if you could afford it, but if you can't afford to go to school, then that's kind of bad.

T: So there's some things he does that make you angry?

C: He's just frustrating. He's like a little kid.

T: He gets angry when you do things right.

C: Right. When I do things the right way, which he knows is the way that I do things, some things that I do are better, but he doesn't . . .

T: He doesn't want to hear it.

C: Yeah, he doesn't want to hear it from me. He just gets mad at me.

T: So if you come across real parental and put a collar around him, it would not go over real well.

C: No.

T: I'm sure you don't feel good when you're not in control.

C: Yeah, I mean totally, totally anxious feeling. I always like to be in control of things in my life, and when I'm not, it bothers me to no end.

T: Well, it's hard when there's such danger out there. Sharks are dangerous. They eat people.

C: *(laugh)* Right, I see him having a real hard time.

T: What he is going through with the suicide in the spring and with two deaths by fire is a lot of danger. It sounds like he's in crisis.

C: Yeah, and I see his girlfriend as not being real, like I love her, she's a very sweet girl, but she's not doing anything good for him. My personal feeling about a relationship is that you should be able to do good things for each other. She's frustrating to me because I don't see her doing anything that I would want a girlfriend to do for my brother.

T: You want her to do some of the things for him that you can't do.

C: Yeah, because I'm not there and someone should do something. And she has the most influence on him of anyone. And when I see her taking a passive role, probably because I'm an aggressive person, that to me is frustrating. And my brother is frustrating because, like, he doesn't get the grades.

T: What do you do when you're a coach and somebody doesn't want to do what they need to?

C: I tell them, "I'm sorry you don't want to do it, you can get out and go tell your parents why you don't want to do it." I just had this problem with this kid last night. He's a very nice kid, but he wants to do things his way. I'm a girl, and he's a boy, so the sexism is already starting (*laugh*). And he's like, "Well, this is the way that it's supposed to be because my dad always tells my mom what to do." And I'm like, "What? This is my little coaching session, and you're going to listen to me." Most of them are having a good time, so they listen to me. There's one boy in the first session and one boy in the second session that don't want to listen. I just made them sit out for 10 minutes, and then they came back in and everything was fine. I don't want them to think I'm mad at them, I just want them to know that they're going to have to listen to me.

T: So you've learned how to deal with kids.

C: Yeah.

T: You've learned how to deal with your dog.

C: Right (*laugh*), anything little (*laugh*).

T: It's a bit difficult, isn't it?

C: Yeah, it's hard with someone that you're on the same level with.

T: You haven't gotten to any issues with your boyfriend yet, but I wonder if you get into some of the same issues with him? These are some of the things that couples get into a lot.

C: Yeah.

T: You talked about him switching to study the way you do.

C: Yeah, but that's good because his grades have improved a lot (*laugh*) since he met me, and I've become a less tense person since I met him.

T: But it sounds like what you're saying is you have this desire to coach and protect and your brother doesn't like it. It's something you have to look at when you choose to do that.

C: Yeah, that's definitely been hard for me.

T: Because you're good at it. It's hard to not take over for everybody.

C: Right, I know. My boyfriend will say, "I love you to death, and I love the things you tell me and I take them to heart, but I can't always do things your way." I was like, "Oops." It's good that he tells me that because sometimes I get caught up in, you know, this is the way it is supposed to go.

T: That's good that he tells you to butt out.

C: Yeah *(laugh)*, he's good at that *(laugh)*.

T: You have to learn what the boundaries are.

C: Yeah, and right now I feel like I'm still trying to learn where to draw the line because no one wants someone who's going to dictate to them.

T: It's a very fine line.

C: Yeah, it is because, like, you want people to know that you care about them, so you want to help them. You want to do what you can do for them, but you don't want them to live their life by you.

COMMENTARY

This client was very talkative and eager to figure out her dream because she had been feeling a great deal of stress. Although she was usually a happy-go-lucky, well-adjusted person, she had been feeling anxious and overwhelmed. She had not been able to put all the pieces together and understand what was making her so tense at the present moment.

She was able to reimmerse herself in the dream, describe the images fully, and associate to each of the images. Her associations quickly revealed the importance of her family. Furthermore, the setting of the dream at the family's summer house where she had just spent a very tense summer with her older brother suggested that her relationship with her brother was troubling her. The images of the puppy and boyfriend suggested that they were also very important to her.

When asked about what the dream meant, she initially thought it had to do with her transition to becoming an adult and recent stresses. Indeed, that may have been part of it, but during this phase I continually but gently confronted her with parts of the dream that didn't fit that interpretation—the fact that there was danger in the dream and that she wasn't able to rescue the faceless man. It is important not to accept the initial interpretation immediately, but to struggle to make the pieces of the dream fit together in an understandable interpretation. As we continually went back to the dream, the situation with the older brother became clearer. I should note that I had no idea what the dream meant when I first heard it; it was only through the exploration of the images that we came to construct what the dream meant for her.

Each dream provides a number of things that could be explored, so therapists have to make choices about what to focus on. I could have probed more about the boyfriend, although she currently seemed to be pretty satisfied about the relationship. I could have probed more about why she felt so responsible for everyone, the number of activities that she was involved in, her relationship with her roommates, and the differences between sharks and puppies. But the energy seemed to be with the older brother, who was possibly represented by the faceless man whom she let be eaten by sharks and the puppy who was out of control. As she talked more, it seemed that the sharks represented the dangers she felt he was being exposed to and that she lacked the ability to protect him from. Although I probed for why she did not rescue the faceless man, she did not seem ready to explore that issue.

If we had had more time, I would have liked to ask her how the different parts of the dream reflected different parts of herself. It would have been fascinating and informative to have her talk about what part of her was like her brother, for example. She was so much into being in total control that it would have been good for her to think about what part of her would have liked to give up. It would also have been interesting to hear what she thought about the part of herself that she just lets die. Perhaps there was a part of herself that she was just letting die at the time.

The action that we came up with was for her to act differently with her brother. Her action was really in terms of not acting—being available for her brother without trying to take over for him. She realized she needed to do some self-talk with herself, as she did with her parents, and tell herself that her brother had to do things on his own. She got a glimmer of some difficulties that she had trying to control everything, although we did not fully explore how she was going to change that. I reminded her that she knew how to deal with kids and puppies and that her boyfriend does not let her control him.

I did not spend as much time as I would have liked on action because we ran out of time (the session was already 90 minutes). We could have used another session to help her work on issues of control. I wish that I had asked her how she would have changed the dream. It would have been interesting to see whether she would have tried to save the faceless guy or would have changed the sharks. Whatever she chose to change would have told us more about her readiness to change.

This client did not seem to need to work on specific behavioral changes in her life at the time. She was generally functioning pretty well. My sense was that she needed to pay more attention to her feelings about her brother and face her lack of being able to control him and that she would then be able to act differently. She seemed to have the skills in her repertoire to act appropriately. But certainly one could have focused on specific behavior changes if one had more time.

This client was easy to work with because she was bright and thoughtful and clearly was feeling stress currently. The dream was an ideal avenue for her to explore her current anxiety because she was not able initially to articulate what was troubling her, but she was able to use the dream to get to the troubling issues. The exploration led directly and quickly to the worry that she was feeling about her brother.

CHAPTER TEN

Individual Therapy with Recurrent Dreams and Nightmares

ECURRENT DREAMS and nightmares represent a major problem for many people. Fifty to 65% of college students reported having had a recurrent dream sometime during their lives (Cartwright & Romanek, 1978; Robbins & Houshi, 1983). In comparison with ordinary dreams, recurrent dreams are more likely to contain only the dreamer and involve being attacked or chased (Robbins & Houshi, 1983). The content of recurrent dreams is often anxious, dysphoric, and conflictual and reflective of unresolved problems (Brown & Donderi, 1986) and the experiential tone is predominantly negative (Cartwright & Romanek, 1978). Furthermore, recurrent dreams most often begin in childhood or adolescence, with only a few beginning in adulthood (Robbins & Houshi, 1983).

Theory and research support the view that recurrent dreams reflect long-standing problems (Coolidge & Bracken, 1984; Robbins & Houshi, 1983; Robbins & Tanck, 1992). Cartwright (1979) viewed the repetitive dream as a sign that some emotionally important concerns have not been addressed adequately in waking life. The current thinking is that recurrent dreams represent ongoing and unacknowledged conflicts in a person's life (Domhoff, 1993). Given that dreams reflect waking conflicts, a recurrent dream probably represents a major issue that the person needs to deal with. Until the dreamer resolves issues in his or her waking life, recurrent dreams often continue. Brown and Donderi (1986) reported that people currently having recurrent dreams scored lower on measures of psychological well-being and reported more negative dream content than people who had recurrent dreams in the past.

Although recurrent dreams often begin at times of stress, such as the death of a loved one, they usually reflect the stress indirectly (e.g., being chased) rather than directly (e.g., the actual death). However, in cases of PTSD, people often dream the exact sequence of events from the traumatic event over and over, making sleep unpleasant and often impossible. Vivid nightmares of combat have been reported for years after the actual event, sometimes occurring after some latency of time (Wilmar, 1982). In fact, recurrent dreams (really nightmares) are one of the defining features of PTSD (Ross, Ball, Sullivan, & Caroff, 1989).

Hartmann (1984) and Kramer, Schoen, and Kinney (1987) discovered several interesting things about the traumatic dreams of Vietnam veterans. In comparison with soldiers who went through similar combat experiences but did not have recurrent traumatic dreams, soldiers who had traumatic dreams were younger, less educated, and more likely to be close with a buddy who was killed or injured in the war (Hartmann, 1984). As the veterans recovered, often through discussion with other veterans who had similar dreams, their dreams slowly began to change and resemble ordinary dreams. When faced with new stressors, however, those who had recovered often relapsed and began having the traumatic dream again.

About 5–10% of children between the ages of 3 and 8 experience disturbing dreams or nightmares at least once a week. The frequency of nightmares declines over age so that most adults have nightmares only about once a year. Cartwright and Lamberg (1992) speculated that our nightmares subside as we grow older because we feel more competent to cope with the world. Hartmann (1984) suggested that some people have had nightmares their whole lives, but others develop nightmares only after some trauma or crisis. He noted that defenselessness is a common thread that runs across all nightmare sufferers, with some having had minimal self-confidence and self-esteem their whole lives and others recently having had a major blow to their self-esteem.

Domhoff (1993) speculated that traumatic dreams serve as a metaphoric expression of our concerns and emotional preoccupations. He further postulated that recurrent dreams are watered-down versions of PTSD dreams and nightmares. Domhoff thought that PTSD dreams, nightmares, and recurrent dreams all reflect preoccupations with stressful waking events. He suggested that traumatic recurrent dreams differ from PTSD dreams, however, in that they are more metaphoric in content rather than being exact repetitions of the stressful experience.

Fortunately, clinical evidence indicates that recurrent dreams and nightmares often disappear when the precipitating problems are resolved (Cartwright, 1979). Hence, working with recurrent dreams and nightmares in individual therapy or dream groups seems advisable.

The following excerpt is presented as an illustration of working with recurrent dreams in individual therapy using the model. The client was a 46-year-old woman who had recently married for the first time.

She had been sexually abused as a child and played the role of the good girl and hero in her family of origin. She served as a nurse in two tours of duty in Vietnam, a situation that seemed to replicate the chaos of her family. Therapy focused on her PTSD that began during the Vietnam War and was reactivated by the Gulf War. In addition, she discussed stresses due to a number of changes during the past year (marriage, moving from her own home to her husband's home in a new area where she had no friends, a new career), dealt with past losses, and examined fears that she had of her husband being injured or killed or of her having a mental breakdown. The therapist was a 33-year-old, advanced male doctoral student in counseling psychology who had a psychodynamic orientation and was trained in the Hill dream interpretation model. This session was the 5th of 12 sessions of a successful case of brief individual therapy conducted for the Diemer et al. (1996) study (see Chapter 12 for more detail about this study). The client and therapist both read the transcript of this session and gave consent for it to be used in this book.

The transcript has been edited to make it shorter and easier to read, but the content of the dialogue has not been altered. The beginnings of the first two stages are indicated so that readers can refer back to the dream interpretation model. C stands for client and T stands for therapist in the transcript.

EXPLORATORY STAGE

The Dream

C: This was a really, excruciatingly hard dream. It was very violent. There were some times that the violence was toward me by me, and sometimes it was like violence toward others.

I remember being at the Vietnam Veterans Wall. I took my scrapbook, which was an old Army issue registry book, olive drab cloth cover. It's one of these books that all of the pages are pasted together. It was used in the Army for keeping things in a generic book that you could use for anything. I made a scrapbook out of it when I was in Vietnam. I kept photos of different patients, evacuation rosters, military pay certificates, which was the money that we used there, and poems that I had written, that others had written. It was a combination of things. It was sort of like the first tour in Vietnam. I was carrying it when my dream starts. I'm standing at the Wall. I'm really distraught. I feel like everything I have worked for, everything that I have done in my life is worthless. I feel so very alone, as though I am the only person that's gone through this, and that there's no one to take care of me, and I've taken care of so many. I feel like I'm being engulfed by all of these memories and by all the really horrible things that went on in Vietnam. I take my book and throw it at the Wall. There's people standing around, and I say, "Take this, take back the memories, I don't want them any more." I'm feeling like the only way I can get past this is to put it in the past, to give it back, and say, "I don't want any part of you anymore, I've had enough, I've had enough, and I don't want any more of this." After throwing the book at the Wall, I say, "Now take the rest of me," and I pull out a gun and shoot myself through the heart. I do that so that nobody can use any more of me, so that they can't use me for a donor. They can't take any more of me, that I've had enough taken. It's like my one last act to at least have some peace.

C: For me the dream felt very real. There were times I really thought that I would act out that dream this summer. It felt so much like (*pause, sniffle, has been crying softly throughout but now it is more obvious*), just being alone was so, so terribly painful. I could see all these other people who had been there were having support, other nurses were having support, and there's none for me. I just felt like I had to keep being stronger, and stronger, and stronger, and ignoring all of the cancer that was crawling up inside me.

T: You just didn't have any more.

C: It was like there was nothing more to give. The last thing I could give was just to make a statement, I guess, that this has been painful. I guess in a way I just didn't know how to cry out for help . . .

T: Mm.

C: . . . Because all my life I've had to do the things myself. Whatever I've gotten I've had to get it myself. It was like something was wrong if you have to go to others to get it. I think that's something I have to really change. From there the dream diverges even more. There's other times I open the door and there's some people at the door that have guns. They're trying to break into my house. Most of the time they're white males, kind of working class, sort of like my father was.

T: Mm.

C: But also they're sort of like the angry young men that you see around so much today. They're yelling things like "bitch" at me. I immediately grab the man's gun, like he's coming in the door, and he's got the gun in his right hand, and I immediately grab his arm and kick out his legs from underneath him at the same time I'm grabbing, and then I stomp on his throat and kill him. When I wake up from the dream I'm like this, like I have been prepared to fight. I've woken up from so many dreams this summer where I'm pulling back my arm to fight . . .

T: Mm.

C: . . . Like I'm prepared to go down fighting. I'm tired of giving in all the time.

T: So it goes both ways this dream? It either goes to you shooting yourself or to this piece about someone coming in the door and you fighting.

C: Yeah, or there's sometimes when I'm killing myself. Another time in the same dream I'm standing in the middle of my house, the one that I finally sold, and I'm standing there just crying, wailing. I feel again so alone, and like I have lost everything that I've worked for, everything that I've tried to do in my life is gone. I don't want somebody else to take it from me. I have a can of gasoline, and I spread it all over the house.

T: Mm.

C: I light the match, and I'm in a circle, and there's gas. I've poured the gasoline all around except for this one circle. I finally light the match and everything starts going up. I'm in the circle, and then I kill myself with a gun. I shoot myself either in the heart or the brain, like to know that it won't be an attempt. The dream diverges again. Just before I light the match, I call the emergency number and I say, "Come to [her address] because there's a donor for you."

T: Mm!

C: As soon as the trucks come up, I don't have gasoline at that time, as soon as the trucks come up and they come to the door, then I shoot myself in the head. I have a note saying, "Take my body, donate the kidneys, donate the heart, donate the this . . . "

T: It's interesting, in the Wall dream it was just what you didn't want to happen.

C: In the Wall dream, it is exactly the opposite. In the Wall dream, it's like I don't want to give any more to Vietnam. It's taken so much from me.

T: Shall we go back and look then at the first one, the Wall dream . . .

C: Yeah.

T: . . . and try to understand that? The way we would do it is to look at each part of the dream, each symbol separately, and try to understand that meaning. Pretend I've never been to Washington and never seen the Wall. I don't know what you mean by the Wall. I'm from another planet. Can you tell me about the Wall, just what does it look like?

C: The Wall is like a giant tombstone. It has like 50,000 names on it. It is black granite that's polished, and you can see yourself in it. It's in the shape of a chevron, which is a military symbol. When you're a private, you have one chevron; when you're a private first class, you get three chevrons. You can walk the length of the wall. You start out where it's like really tiny, it's a point of the chevron, and then you walk to the higher point in the middle, and then it bends and goes back to a smaller point.

T: Can you tell me about the personality of the Wall?

C: It's sort of like a monument.

T: If it's a person, what is its personality?

C: I want to say peace, but it's not really that. The people that are dead no longer feel the pain that they went through. But it reflects all the pain that everybody has brought to it. It reflects it back to them.

T: This person is in pain?

C: Well this person is at peace so that people that come to look at it get their own pain reflected back to them, that sometimes we get some of the peace reflected back too. The first time I saw it, I went there on my 20th anniversary of having gone to Vietnam, and I felt very much at peace in a way because I had come sort of full circle from where I'd left and come back. It's kind of like 50,000 stories on it. Everybody who comes finds a different story for themselves. I know a lot of the stories of the people whose faces are reflected there. There's the names of three men who died in a helicopter crash because they couldn't be rescued by this one sergeant. I know the pain of what this man talked about, about not being able to rescue three men and how for years and years he's held that pain.

T: So the Wall has a lot of stories to tell.

C: Yeah, a lot more than 50,000.

T: Is it peaceful with the stories? Is it sad? Is it a sad Wall?

C: It can be anything, it changes, it depends upon the reflection that's there. The day I went in the dream was a painful one because it was drawing so much from me. I couldn't see my reflection in the wall anymore. I was having so much pain but I was invisible to the source of it, just like I was invisible in my family. It's like it was taking over too much of my life.

T: In the dream it was taking over too much?

C: Yeah, that's why I threw my memories at it. Let it at least swallow them up instead of me. I thought maybe if I could give back my memories.

T: Mm.

C: But then I thought, too, if I left my memories at the Wall, then there would be people that would come and they'll take apart those memories. They will take the military pay certificates out of the book because those are souvenirs, they could sell them for a price. They'll take the pictures. They take all the different things. They would rip them apart from me.

T: Even though this is a dream?

C: Yeah, I think at the time that I thought this is when I pulled out the gun and killed myself.

T: So you threw it at the Wall and it bounced off the Wall?

C: Yeah.

T: It didn't absorb it?

C: No, it kind of scattered the pages around. There were people that came up and then took parts of it because it would be worth money. It was like my memories. It was like the yard sale. It was like the house. And nobody said, "Thank you."

T: No acknowledgment.

C: No. It's kind of like give me more, give me more, and keep giving me more, and finally I gave everything that I could. To me the only way that I could give that much was to end the pain for myself. I wished I could feel good about my role of being there, yet I feel so bad about it. It's as though there are some names on the Wall that shouldn't be there, that if we would have done this or we would have done that. I think we did the best we could with the knowledge we had at the time, but I don't feel good.

T: So as hard as you try and as much as you worked, you still weren't able to fix it.

C: Yeah. It was like if I wouldn't have gone to the helicopter party the night before, the one night for getting away from the war, maybe I would have caught this or caught that or something would have changed.

T: So instead of feeling good about what you did, the individual lives that you saved, people that you helped and comforted, it's blame for the pieces that you missed.

C: Yeah, I think so. But I know that there's a name on the Wall of a man who shouldn't have died. Yet it wasn't just me that missed a clue. There were several surgeons and a lot of other nurses who missed a clue.

T: Tell me how many names on the Wall are people that should have died.

C: I don't think any of those should have.

T: Yeah, but you are assuming the blame for the one that you think you let go.

C: It's just that I always felt that I could have done better. Sometimes it's like I judge myself on knowledge that we learned 5 years later.

T: Mm.

C: You go back and judge yourself on, "If we would have done this, if we would have done that."

T: Mm.

C: There's some men whose names I don't know. I don't even remember their first names. I remember exactly what they looked like, like this one soldier, but I don't know his name. I don't remember the name of this guy with 100% third-degree burns that they dropped off in the ward to let die. They left me with him. Everybody else supported each other, but they forgot the main nurse who had to talk to him, take care of him. I couldn't tell him that they had decided to shut off his fluids because there was no hope for him. He didn't know he was dying. He couldn't see because his body was bloated up, he was completely burned, and his eyes were swollen shut, so he at least couldn't see what his body looked like. Nobody thought of me, they just assumed that I'd take care of it. But yet the chaplain had support, and the doctor had support, and everybody else had support, but nobody ever supported me on that (*crying openly*).

T: Nobody took care of your pain.

C: Nobody even recognized that it would be difficult for me. Yet I had to go ahead and take care of him. I did the best I could. That night they told me to give him as much morphine as he needed to stay out of pain. I could see as time went on he kept getting in more and more pain. The last time that he was groaning, we started to get casualties back in through the emergency room, so I wasn't going to have the time to talk with him anymore. He had started lapsing into a bit of a coma, but he was starting to groan. His respirations were where normally you wouldn't give the morphine, but he was groaning and in pain. It's like do you hold off on the morphine until his respirations come up or do you give the morphine because he is in pain? I gave him the morphine because I knew he was in pain and he was groaning. He died 15 minutes after the last morphine I gave him. In some ways I felt like I had killed him, and in another way I felt like I had freed him. I had a nightmare that night . . .

T: Mm hmm.

C: . . . Where I woke up screaming saying, "Give me 3 days, that's all I have of my life, but give me my life, give me the rest of my life." We had never discussed that the best we could give him was 3 days before he would lapse into a coma. If we gave him fluids and we did all the things that we'd do normally for a burn victim, we could give him 3 days. But we didn't even give him that. I took away the rest of his life. I didn't give him a choice in it, ask him what he wanted to do with the rest of his life.

T: What do you imagine he would have done with his 3 days?

C: I didn't know whether it would have been so painful for him or if he would have been able to at least talk to his family by way of a recording or something to do some unfinished business. At least he would have had the choice. I don't know where his name is on the Wall . . .

T: Mm.

C: . . . But I know the story. I can still feel the story.

T: Sounds like it. I can feel it. It's very powerful. Tell me why were you angry at the Wall.

C: Because Vietnam keeps coming back. In all my dreams this summer I would fade in to one part of the dream and then fade in to Vietnam. It was like it keeps recycling. I thought that it was over for me.

T: And now it's back.

C: It's been back since the Gulf War, and it's never left again.

T: Mm.

C: I'm ready for it to leave. Yet there is another part of me that says this was a part of me, that it changed a lot of my life. But I'm still angry because of these veterans that hold up these signs that say, "Homeless veteran, dejected, rejected, and so forth." It's like they're saying, "Take care of me, you didn't take care of me back then, you have to keep taking care of me the rest of my life." I want to stop taking care of people that need to take care of themselves. On the Wall there's the name of the man who I gave morphine to. He went up in an airplane to take pictures, and the plane crashed and he died from third-degree burns.

T: Mm.

C: He wasn't out on a mission or combat. (*pause*) It's like the Wall keeps saying, "Take care, take care, take care."

T: The Wall is telling you to take care of them?

C: (*sigh*) In some ways.

T: So fix these 50,000, fix the war, fix the pain.

C: And don't worry about your own.

T: Put it aside.

C: Yeah, like, "We want this, we want that, we want." There's one part of me that feels like there's names that aren't on the Wall because of me and my friends and all the things we did, but there's a lot of the names on the Wall.

T: So you worked, and you put aside your pain, and you still aren't able to fix it.

C: Yeah, I went back to Vietnam a second time, and it was during the second time that this man, this experience, happened. The first time was when this man died who had been on the respirator for about 15 days. The doctor said that the man's body just couldn't take it anymore, that he was worn out, and treatment was discontinued. Later we found out that the cause of death was a ruptured spleen and that if he had been taken back to surgery, he would most likely have been saved. I went back to Vietnam because of him, kind of to find my own salvation, I guess?

T: To save him this time.

C: To make up for it. Yet here's this other man who there's no way I could have saved, nobody could have saved him. I know that, but it's like I expected more from myself. I expected to know all the things that could go wrong. His death helped in that I was able to help other people to die well at least and help finish up the business and everything, to lead them into a peaceful sort of death, not by euthanasia, but by having the courage to sit and talk with somebody who is dying.

T: Doing some of the things that you wanted to do with him.

C: Yeah, but this summer I got engulfed by so many things, and the Wall was there. It's a good enough place to take it out on.

T: So the Wall symbolized everything, all your failures in fixing the war.

C: And fixing myself. It's as much fixing myself, like the person that I am today is because of me. I have pulled myself up out of a horrible situation at home, out of a horrible war, again and again. I've not led the standard life, you know? Everything that I have, all that I know right now, is because I've sought out the answers for myself. I've tried to learn. Yet I'm finding it's not enough. I think the overwhelming loneliness has gotten to me this summer. I think it's because of all the changes that happened.

T: Mm.

C: It's been really, really difficult. There's some changes that I wanted to happen that didn't. I wanted to be able to finally say, "Vietnam is a part of me, but it's a past part of me. My family is a part of me, but it's a past part of me, the way the family was." I don't want to go back to what that family is.

T: Mm.

C: I don't want to go back to what Vietnam was. Yet I think that most war veterans run into the same sort of problem. There is something about the war that just doesn't end. It just plays on and on forever.

T: If the war was a continuation of something for you, what would it be?

C: I think it's like I'm in a war zone now. Our country is becoming very much like a war zone, and I don't think a lot of people notice it. It's not that much different than Vietnam in some ways.

T: Mm.

C: We'll probably have as much body count as what we had in Vietnam, I suspect. Only our weapons are not just AK47's and M16's, but they're cars, and they're drugs, and they're handguns, and things like that. Just the way people treat each other, it's as though they're in a war. It's as though they're losing their civilness.

T: Manners get put aside in wars.

C: Yeah.

T: Other persons' feelings get put aside. Nobody acknowledges too much going on.

C: Yeah.

T: No time. Gotta get.

C: But the war's different in a way, in that everybody who was working there, at least the first time I was at the war . . .

T: Mm.

C: . . . There was a comradeship. We're all in it together. After you had worked your 12-hour shift a day, you didn't go off to the movies or to this or that. You went home, and then you got up the next day 12 hours later, and you worked for another 12–13 hours, and you did that 6 days a week on good weeks.

INSIGHT STAGE

T: (*deep breath*) Can we go back to the dream real quick and try to make sense of some of the symbols there and see if we can understand what the dream is telling you, if there's a message in the dream? I mean there's a real obvious piece to it. You made some associations to the Wall in your stories. The Wall seems to really symbolize for you, as I'm sure it does for a lot of people, the pain of the war, and for you a lot of the failures, that you blame yourself in a lot of ways for things that you couldn't fix. It's like an open wound, isn't it?

C: It gets better each time I go back. I think that it heals a little bit more, but it's not completely healed. Sometimes it festers, and it's got to be opened up again. I think this summer it was festering.

T: Mm. You couldn't close it.

C: It's just not closing. I'm ready for it to.

T: The element that I picked up on was a sense of giving up—I can't do it anymore, I can't fight this wound anymore. No matter how I try, no matter how I work, I can't close it. Does that ring . . . ?

C: I think so. It's like the frustration I feel, only much more magnified, when I'm working on a module in a [computer] program . . .

T: Mm.

C: . . . And it keeps doing the wrong thing. I get really frustrated, like I'm in a loop and can't get out.

T: Mm.

C: . . . That's kind of the same way, only much, much more magnified. It's like I'm in a loop. I'm doing something, and I'm not finding the way of breaking out of it to end it so I can go on to the next part.

T: So you're trapped.

C: Yeah. I thought I had gotten out of it back when I lived in another city. I felt at peace with Vietnam for 2 years there. Then the Gulf War came.

T: Mm.

C: It's like I went right back into it. It's even harder right now, but I think it's partly because of all of the loss. It's not just the loss of all of the men's lives, but it's all the loss that I've gone through this summer.

T: Is there a connection to your family too?

C: Yeah, like with my sister. When she started to give me excuses again, I didn't know what to say.

T: Mm hmm.

C: I had told her in black and white what to say.

T: Mm.

C: "I'm sorry," was all that she had to say. When she started speaking to me, it was almost as though it just touched me off. I don't want to be in this loop anymore. I don't want to be in this family as it was.

T: Is there a person before your sister that it was like? That same kind of frustration?

C: My father, the church that I went to, some old relationships were like that in a way, in that I kept giving, and giving, and giving, and not getting anything back.

T: And what is this dream telling you?

C: (*sigh*) If I stay in the course that I'm on, the dream might come true.

T: Mm.

C: The dream really frightened me a lot this summer. We do have a handgun at home I bought a few years ago when there was an outbreak of rape. I unloaded the gun because I wanted to have to load the gun if I did anything. That would give me at least thinking about it.

T: Mm.

C: When I went to work on the house, I left the gun at home because I didn't want to take the chance—this is just too tempting.

T: Yeah.

C: It scares me too much because it's almost as though if I can't get past the pain, then I don't think I want to continue. As long as I can keep on going, even if I go back down for a bit, if I crawl up maybe another inch from where I was, that's okay.

T: Mm.

C: But if I'm sliding down and I don't have any chance of getting back up, that's not so much okay. That's not how I want my life.

T: So the dream is telling you to get past these things or else.

C: I think it's telling me too that you have to look at these things and you have to start dealing with them again.

T: But you are.

C: Yeah. I think that's why the dreams started. I still get elements of the violent dream of people trying to attack and I attack back. I wake up in the middle of the night and I'm frightened, and then that scares me some.

T: It's a very scary thing, horribly scary.

C: Yeah, I don't want to be in a situation where I'm having to fight for my life all the time.

T: Yeah.

C: That's a war zone. I've had enough war zones.

T: I'll say, one war zone after another.

C: I always said that my first tour in Vietnam was a breeze because I had come from a worse war zone than what Vietnam was.

T: Right. Well, we've talked about a lot of important stuff today.

C: Yeah.

T: I think it's important for us to come back to the war, what happened in your family, and what happened in your house when you sold it and the stuff in it. These are all sort of open wounds that are sucking you in to fix . . .

C: Mm hmm.

T: . . . Them. You just can't fix it and make it better, and that has absolutely sucked you in and overwhelmed you. Those are very powerful feelings.

C: I think what's overwhelming me is not getting the acknowledgment. For me, that is the hardest part.

T: Yeah.

C: It's like I'm down and nobody seems to notice, like I'm just flat out in the dirt and people are walking by.

T: Yeah, right over you.

C: Yeah, and that's sort of the family, I think.

T: Mm hmm. I think we should try to spend a little bit of time, go back and understand what happened in your family . . .

C: Mm hmm.

T: . . . Because I see a connection between the family, the two service duties in the War, and what's happened in the last year . . .

C: Yeah.

T: . . . Giving away your house and all that. I think it's real important for us to understand how they are all connected.

C: Yeah, I think so too.

COMMENTARY

This client reported a very troubling recurrent dream about committing suicide at the Vietnam Memorial Wall. Although technically the dream was not a PTSD dream because it was not an exact replica of a specific traumatic event, the dream was clearly related to trauma this woman had experienced as a nurse during the Vietnam War.

The client was very talkative and quickly got into exploring the images of her dream. The therapist gently guided her and generally allowed her to explore the images and themes in her own way rather than specifically structuring the process for the client to do associations to each image. The client reported at the follow-up that she felt that the therapist could feel her pain and that his empathy made it easier to talk about this violent dream. The exploration of the images of the dream (e.g., the Wall) naturally led into insight about what the dream meant (i.e., that current events and the recent Gulf War had stirred up memories of abuse from childhood and violence from the Vietnam War and that she was in danger of fragmenting or committing suicide from the stress). The therapist was very gentle and supportive of the client, who obviously was emotionally wrought up about her memories. The therapist allowed the client to progress at her own speed and did not force her to follow the structure of the dream interpretation model rigidly given that she obviously needed to cathart. Given her fragility, the client probably could not have handled a more directive therapist.

Although the therapist helped the client progress through the first two stages of the model, they did not get as far as the Action Stage. The client was very talkative and somewhat controlling and often digressed from the dream (many of these sections were deleted to make for easier reading). The client also had not incorporated enough insight to have any action be readily apparent. Thus, the client probably was not ready for the Action Stage. The therapist could easily have spent another session discussing the associations and delving into the memories of the abusive early family situation.

The therapist might have been able to stimulate the Action Stage by asking the client to say how she would have liked to change the dream if she could have it be any way she wanted. My own fantasy is that the client would have said that she would have liked to have gone to the Wall with her family and asked them to listen to her stories of her childhood and the war. Perhaps in her revised dream, her family might ask her for forgiveness.

The therapist later indicated to me that the dream interpretation was helpful for the client in that it was the first time that she was able to tune into her affect during the treatment. The structure of the dream interpretation seemed useful for this client, even though she resisted having the therapist take too much control. The client made it clear that she wanted to be taken care of; fortunately, the therapist was able to provide her with appropriate support and reassurance. During the remainder of the therapy, the therapist and client repeatedly returned to the images raised during this dream interpretation, particularly the image that the client was "used up" and had no more to give.

The client clearly remembered the dream and the dream interpretation when I asked her permission 2 years later to use the transcript of the session for this book. She reported that she had been to the Wall a number of times and that she had recently had a good, long talk with her mother about her traumatic experiences. She felt good that her mother had been able to listen to her and comfort her. She knew that she still had more work to do, but it seemed as though she was coping better with the childhood traumas, the war experiences, and her present marital situation.

CHAPTER ELEVEN

Dream Groups

DREAM GROUPS are an exciting modality for working with dreams (Cushway & Sewell, 1992; Shuttleworth-Jordan, Saayman, & Faber, 1988; Taylor, 1983; Ullman, 1979, 1987, 1993; Ullman & Zimmerman, 1979). A primary feature of structured dream groups is that dreams are the topic of each session. Ideally, groups are structured so that only one person presents a dream at each session, thus ensuring that an adequate amount of time is set aside for delving into each dream. Furthermore, scheduling only one dream per session prevents the more vocal members from getting all the attention and the more reticent people from not getting to be focal member.

Another major feature of this approach as applied to groups is that all group members project their associations, insights, and possible actions onto the dream as if the dream were their own (Ullman, 1979, 1987; Ullman & Zimmerman, 1979). By having all group members project onto an individual's dream, everybody stays involved and learns something new for themselves. In addition, the dreamer gets many different viewpoints about how other people respond to his or her dream. The dreamer is free to explore whether the other viewpoints fit, opening up the possibility to explore aspects that may have been out of awareness. The dreamer, of course, always has the final say in determining which aspects of the dream interpretation fit for him or her. Respect for the dream, and dreamer, is a key aspect of this approach (see also Ullman & Zimmerman, 1979).

Dream groups can be particularly powerful when organized around a shared experience such as divorce (e.g., Falk & Hill, 1995). Because clients have had similar experiences, they are likely to have experienced similar feelings. Hence, if one person is blocking, another can help him or her with the feelings. Additionally, it is sometimes easier to examine one's own problems at a distance through thinking about someone else who has a similar problem.

Groups using this model have a dual purpose. First, they aim to help the individual dreamer understand his or her dream, using the entire group as cotherapists. A second aim is to have those members whose dreams are not being presented project their own issues onto the dream that is presented. The assumption behind this approach is that people can project onto anything, but whatever each person projects reflects his or her own thought structure. Thus, everyone in the group could have different associations to an image because they have all had different past experiences, and they all have different schemata. Thus, each person can benefit from examining his or her thoughts about another person's dream.

The format for dream groups is slightly modified from the overall approach to dream interpretation presented in Chapter 4. Groups usually are scheduled for a minimum of 90 minutes, preferably 2 hours, to provide enough time to do justice to each dream interpretation. During the first session, therapists provide an overview of the model, giving group members an outline of the three stages so that they can participate more fully. The general structure of each session in a dream interpretation group is to begin with a brief go-round in which all group members describe current thoughts and feelings and how they have used what they learned in the last group session during the week. After the go-round, one member then tells a dream, which becomes the focus for the remainder of the group session. The dreamer is then asked to explore the dream by using feelings, associations, linkages to waking life, and by working with conflicts in the dream, with the whole group acting in a therapeutic manner (e.g., clarifying, asking questions, reflecting feelings). After the dreamer has responded to the Exploration Stage, each group member very briefly talks about his or her feelings, associations, and linkages to the images. The dreamer then needs to be given a chance to respond and say which things fit for him or her. The group then moves to the Insight Stage, with the group helping the dreamer arrive at possible interpretations to the dream at the various levels. Again, the group members each say what the dream would mean if it were theirs, with the dreamer once more having the final say about which added pieces of interpretation fit for him- or her. The group then helps the dreamer think about action steps, with other group members again indicating what action they would take if the dream were theirs. In a final go-round, each group member discusses what he or she has learned for him or herself from the dream interpretation.

The task of the therapists (or cotherapists) is to guide the group through the stages. They need to monitor the group to make sure that the focus stays on the focal member but that every group member has a chance to talk without dominating the group. When groups are stuck, therapists can offer their own associations, insights, or actions "as if" the dreams were theirs. They need to challenge the focal dreamer to try out other levels of interpretation or action, especially if the group is reticent about confronting the dreamer. They also must work on making the group cohesive so that the members feel that they can share their thoughts and feelings safely and feel support from the group. The therapists do not let any one group member dominate the time, they try to encourage the quiet members to talk, and they stop group members when they become hostile or nasty to other group members.

Therapists need to stress the ground rules of confidentiality and indicate that people can stop whenever they want without being pushed to reveal more than is comfortable. One of the potential problems with dreams is that people often reveal things about themselves without being aware of it. Because people cannot always know when a dream will reveal "forbidden material," clients are allowed to stop the process if they need to. As in individual therapy, groups often require some time together before members feel comfortable revealing deep feelings. Dream interpretation can lead quickly to deep feelings, so therapists need to monitor client readiness carefully. Monitoring of progress is also necessary to ensure that clients are able to deal with the dream material uncovered in the group process. Sometimes it is useful to encourage clients to be in individual therapy as well as in a group to work on identified problems so that the group can stay focused on dreams.

The following transcript is from the fifth of eight sessions of a group conducted for the Falk and Hill (1995) study. The cotherapists were female doctoral students in counseling psychology. The clients were five adult women adjusting to recent separation or divorce. The transcript begins after the initial go-round when the dreamer retells her dream.

The transcript has been edited to make it shorter and easier to read, but the content of the dialogue has not been altered. The dreamer and both cotherapists read the transcript and consented to have it reprinted in this book. I have indicated where each of the three stages begins so the reader can refer back to the dream interpretation model. The client who presented a dream is D; the other clients are C2, C3, C4, and C5; the therapists are T1 and T2.

EXPLORATION STAGE

The Dream

I have these two beautiful kittens, but I don't know how I got them. I have a feeling they were given to me, but I don't know who gave them to me. They're not just kittens, they're a strange animal that's both a kitten and a snake from Egypt. They took the form of two very large cobra snakes, the ones that have the big head. I was upstairs at a house that I don't recognize. For some reason the snake was following me around; it was real quick. I was more annoyed than frightened by it. I wanted it to leave me alone, but I was scared to run away or make sudden motions because I thought it would strike at me. So everywhere I went in a room, the snake would follow me, and a cat would appear next to me. I was getting real frustrated. At one point, I thought the snakes were afraid of water. In the middle of the room was a tub and a hose on the ground, so I turned on the water and stood in the water. The snake kept trying to get in close to me again, and it would recoil back. Then the water started going away. The snake started coming in again, so I turned on the hot water harder. There seemed to be water all over the floor. At that point I was like, "I'm going to hurt the snake," because I had hot water. So I turned it off and left the room. The door of the room was one of those glass doors with the wooden border. I shut the door on the snake's face and went downstairs. It headbutted the door and got through and came out after me again. I keep having these images like it's going real quick across the floor. So I went downstairs, and my younger brother was there, and I said, "It's driving me crazy, I can't get the snake away from me." He said, "All it wants to do is get close to you, and if you would let it close to you it would be okay." So I said, "Fine," and these two snakes came over. I just let them get close to me, and they turned back into these two little calico kittens. They were really cute and kept snuggling against me. It wasn't like I felt real tender towards them, but I felt like all I had to do was not be afraid of them and they would be okay, they wouldn't hurt me. The kittens were really going up against me, and one was having me rub its belly. But then I thought, "I can't handle it, I can't have these cats around me all the time." So I thought I would let them out in the woods, and they can turn into snakes. Then I thought, "No, I can't do that, they would come after me." Then I went to my office and posted a sign for a man to get these cats. I decided that they were really men's pets because men like snakes.

T1: Is there any feeling to the end of your dream?

D: No. The whole time I was thinking about how I had to get rid of these cats. They're really cute cats, but I couldn't handle them. There was something with the snakes too. They were too changeable, I guess. The reason I wanted to get rid of them was not that I didn't like the kittens, it was because I didn't know when they would turn into snakes again. I thought, "I can't handle it, a man could handle this kind of pet better because they wouldn't be afraid of snakes, so that's someone who would want this kind of pet." I wasn't disgusted or anything. It was just like I don't know when these are going to become snakes, because I didn't like them when they were snakes.

T1: So your sense was that it was going to work that you posted this sign?

D: Yeah. I know what the sign was about. When I moved to another place and couldn't bring my two cats, I got rid of them by posting a sign in my office, and a woman called and took my two cats away. That was pretty sad, traumatic. But I know that's probably where the posting of the sign came from. I was also posting it to girlfriends to give it to their boyfriends as presents.

T2: Do you have a picture of the sign? What does it look like?

D: It was just handwritten on a white piece of paper, something about a great animal for a man. I just didn't feel like it was an animal for me. It wasn't just like snakes turned into cats. It was harder to explain. In my dream it was one animal, just sometimes it was a snake and sometimes a cat.

C4: There were two of them?

D: There were two of them in the beginning. This one snake kept following me around. Then at the end it was two cats again.

C5: Were the cats the same color?

D: Yeah, there were two really little calico cats with big blue eyes. In my dream I thought I had to get rid of them right away because they were only 2 weeks old. People like kittens, and they would take them right away. But that's impossible, you can't give away 2-week-old cats, but in my mind they were 2 weeks old. They were really tiny.

C2: You were in a shower?

D: It must have been a tub because he was trying to come up on the side.

C2: I thought the protective part was interesting because when the snake was chasing you, I was afraid.

D: He was chasing me, but when he came up he never harmed me. You know how cobras move, he would just come up next to me and move like that.

C2: Do you have an image or picture?

D: It was almost cartoonish. They race across the floor and come up by me. I was scared of it, it was awful, frustrating, like, "Get the hell away from me and just leave me alone."

T2: What level of being scared?

D: The scare was that if I move too quickly, it's going to strike me, kill me, or poison me.

T2: Because that's its nature, not because it wants to?

D: Right, that's its nature. I never got the impression it was trying to harm me, but it had the potential of being dangerous. It wouldn't leave me alone. It followed me everywhere, and I didn't know what it wanted.

T2: So you were more aggravated.

D: I was more aggravated, scared too, but more aggravated.

T1: When you were saying that your reaction was, "I can't handle it and a man could handle it better," can you say more about what handling means?

D: It was fine when they were kittens, but I couldn't handle the fact that any moment it might turn back into a snake. I don't think a man could handle it any better. It was like the kittens were very demanding. The whole animal is very demanding on me and for my attention. But mainly I thought it was a man's animal because of the snake part.

C4: So the one snake turned into two kittens and turned back into one snake.

D: I only remember one snake, but I just assumed there were two snakes because there was two kittens. I only remember one snake following me around. But there were two distinct kittens.

C3: I remember you saying something about the other snake would come in. You mentioned two snakes.

D: Did I?

C2: Yeah.

D: There was always one snake near me. There was one snake bugging the hell out of me. I don't know where the other snake was at the time.

T2: When you're talking about handling, which of your emotions was getting in the way of handling it?

D: My initial feeling is not so much the fear as they're demanding. But that doesn't make sense to me why I would think a man would handle it better. I mean my feeling in the dream was that it was a snake. That was why I thought it was a man's pet.

T2: So which was more demanding—when it was a snake or when it was a kitten?

D: They were both demanding in different ways. The snake was demanding because it followed me everywhere and was there, and I didn't know what the hell it wanted. The reason I couldn't handle the kittens is that they were really affectionate and they were all over me. But if I didn't want them to do that, they were trying to turn into snakes again. That's what I couldn't handle, that if I put them down they would turn into snakes again.

C4: What's going on in your life right now in terms of your personal life? You said that you were dating somebody and you were trying to resolve that situation?

D: It's interesting, I was talking about my dream to a friend last night, and I talked a lot about my mother. So first I was like the snake is my mother. But when I was describing it to a woman I work with today, I was saying, "He, he, he." The snake was a he, so it can't be my mother.

She doesn't have the qualities of the animal. There is something—I'm trying to end a relationship, and I just do not feel like ending it.

T2: Why don't we go on to doing the associations. Pick one or two elements of the dream and associate to them.

D: The two things that are significant are obvious images. I don't know why they are related because they are two opposite animals, but what comes to mind with snakes is very penile, just long and skinny, especially a cobra I guess just in terms of exotic, scary, mysterious, something I don't want to get mad, very, very dangerous. When I think of a cobra, it's mesmerizing. For a kitten, I love cats, so kittens are warm and fuzzy, innocent and sweet and cute, furry.

T2: Are the kittens in your dream associated to those specific kittens?

D: Same thing, but very demanding, but they are still adorable, and they have the noses and tongues and kept kissing me. They made me really happy.

T1: What can you associate to that demanding feeling?

D: Trapped, closed in, depressed, just can't get away from the guilt.

T1: Can you say more about the guilt? What that has to do with demanding?

D: Well, when I think of demanding, I think of my mother. I have a hard time saying no when people make demands on me. Even when I don't want to do something, a lot of times I do it because I feel guilty if I don't do it. That's sort of the feeling with the cats too. I didn't have an option to let them go, to push them away. Even if I did, they would turn around and be snakes and still be around me, except this time they would be dangerous.

T1: It sounded like there was a realization that these were a man's pet and these should be given to a man.

D: Well, it wasn't like it was given, it was like maybe a man would take this away from me. I didn't know if anyone would take them. I was worried that I would be stuck with them. But I thought if anybody would want them, a man would.

T1: So there was no guilt that you were trying to give them away?

D: There was no time for guilt because I was very desperate to get rid of these cats. So the guilt hadn't come, more like desperation.

T1: Are there any other images in the dream that feel especially vivid?

D: It's extremely vivid when I shut the snake in the door and it headbutted it open and came downstairs. I was like, "I can't believe this snake headbutted the door open and got down here after me." That was probably the strongest image to me. I couldn't believe the snake could get the door open.

C4: You watched it do it because it was a glass door?

D: Yeah, I just couldn't believe that the snake headbutted the door open. It didn't break it. It just forced it open and was persistent.

T1: Can you associate to the snake at that point?

D: He was extremely determined. He was going to get to me or whatever he wanted, butt his head against the door, extremely determined and focused. That's a pretty wild image for a snake to be headbutting the door open. After that I was like, "I can't get away from this snake." That's when my brother said, "Give him what he wants and it will turn out okay."

C2: Is the snake as big as you or half as tall as you?

D: When it goes across the thing, it's just like a fairly small size of snake, but when it snipes at me once, I remember I'm sitting down and it was up here, the head was like up here (*hand up high*). The kittens were tiny.

C4: Do you often ask your brother for advice?

D: No, the only reason I think my brother was in my dream is because I have seen him recently, and I talked about him a lot last night, and of all my family my brother is the most centered and has his act together. I don't dream about him a lot, but I did talk about him often.

C4: That he had his stuff together and would be the one in the family that you most likely would ask?

D: I never asked him for advice because I always thought of him as my younger brother. He's only 2 years younger, but as I learn more about him as an adult, I admire him a lot. I like the person he's become.

T1: Can each of the rest of you give an association to one of the images as if this dream had been your own?

C4: Snake, cobra, I just get this sense of personality about a cobra snake, mesmerizing, laid back and cool, but deadly. I'm specifically associating to the cobra because it can also be friendly and has a real personality. I feel the same way about kittens. They're wonderful, cuddly, demanding, and have their own personality. Kittens and cats are completely different in my mind. Kittens are dependent and demanding, a source of great joy and stupid things. Kittens do things like run into walls and shake their heads and come back for more, just a sense of adventure. I think in terms of adventure for snakes too.

C5: As I'm listening I'm getting kind of a general impression of this good versus evil power struggle. It's funny you should mention snakes. The Freudian interpretation would have to be sex. When I was an undergraduate, snaking was a term for sexual intercourse. There's no way you would know that, but it just brought back the memory of that. I was trying to think of some other possible interpretation. First I thought of India and

Pakistan because cobras live there. Then I remembered the Garden of Eden. I know the cobra wasn't the snake in the Garden of Eden, but apparently there was a snake there. If you believe in stories of snakes being the embodiment of all evil, and all evil descended from civilization since then, I get this sense that evil is following you around and you're trying to get rid of it. You're a good-hearted person, you're not trying to invite evil into your life. It's healthy to get rid of evil that can't be expunged completely. Also, count me in the column of cat lovers. Cats are the most precious thing I can think of.

D: They were very happy. They were kissing me all over. And they were just so joyful that I let them get close to me.

C5: Most cats love that way of attention to them. Rub their necks and bellies and kiss their noses, and they're innocent and delightful. They're harmless, helpless, almost like human babies in that respect.

T1: I really hate snakes, and I was really hoping you wouldn't have snakes. This particular snake, it didn't remind me of my difficulties with them, I was just struck by the power of this snake because it's poisonous and unpredictable and so determined—the incredible image of it butting against the door. Also, it's very male to me. When you were talking, I was thinking about the image of a top of a penis. But the maleness I was thinking of is more the kind of power, a football player, violent and incredibly strong. The kittens I thought of in the context of this really powerful snake, your reaction to it; I thought of it as a power struggle. If you try to meet it head on in that same way with the door, it doesn't work. If you decide you're not afraid of it and welcome it, let it be close to you, it would be kittens, not scary, not male, not powerful. It's you becoming empowered by dealing with that power differently. I was struck by the demandingness, always have to be around, and yes cute, but you can't tell them to go away, you're tired of them, take care of yourself for a day. They're always there, they're needing you and want to get close to you.

C2: I had the same association, it's a very big, powerful evil. India for me is exotic, kind of dirty. It's a culture I'm not attracted to. I was put off by it very much. Most of the people I work with are Indian. It's funny because I love them, they're really smart, but it's also true that coming from a culture with castes, they're demanding in a way that's very hard to live with. So all this demanding stuff really ties in for me with this image of India.

D: Yeah, I don't know if it's significant, but I've traveled through India. It was a big experience for me. I don't know if it ties into this image, but I would agree with you. India's very male dominant to the women and children.

C2: I don't like cats, and I especially don't like kittens. I see them as really demanding. You don't get a lot back. You pet them, and they claw you. The only thing I do like about them is that you get a neat smell sometimes from kittens, and they're nice and soft. But the whole business that all these things are controlling you I didn't like.

D: I have a funny image too, but I can't remember clearly. I pushed one of the kittens away, and it did claw me. It didn't hurt, but it was hanging there. I couldn't push him away.

C2: I was very taken when you said you were trying to interpret this to your mother as being some demanding presence that's dangerous to get rid of, because mine's that way too. It's true that you have the say about how you react, to make your decisions and all that, but when you have this astonishingly dangerous person retaliating for what you've done, it's very hard to think of yourself as being in control, so I loved that interpretation.

T2: For me I'm thinking about this snake, I got less of a sense of danger and more of this ever-present worry type of thing of something just hanging around. I was thinking of a rubber-band type of thing where it keeps coming back, it's like attached to you and you can't push it away.

D: Even though I wasn't scared per se, I knew if I made the wrong move it would strike me, it would hurt me.

T2: I was thinking about kittens and how they chase their tails and no matter how much they would try to run away from them, they're always there. I also was thinking about snakes. You mentioned Egypt and associating Egyptian snakes with knowledge and wisdom, and so that there is this knowledge that is in the snake. I was associating that also cats always have a sort of secretive knowledge—that's something I would associate with cats. I have a kitten who wakes me up at 6 o'clock in the morning, whether my daughter wakes me up or not, so my association with that is of demanding—even though you're wonderful, go away. I want to keep pushing the cat out of my life at that time of morning. And the frustration of not being able to train it to fit in with my needs and my lifestyle and my routine, so that's probably it for me.

C3: I think from what I read, I symbolize both cats and snakes as an Egyptian type of thing. I'm glad you didn't hurt the snake, but when it comes right up (*motions like a cobra*), I just had the feeling, "Get the hell out of my face."

D: Well that's exactly what I thought, "Get the fuck away from me." I didn't know what it wanted either.

C3: Trapped was a good word you used, that's the same way I feel when he was sitting there going like this (*motions like a cobra*), "Get away." I think on the other extreme that kittens can be as independent as heck, to the point of almost manipulation of, "You are going to pet me when I want you to, if I want to be held I'll let you know, you don't let me know."

So it's a form of control, and this thing is controlling you because you are afraid that if you do something it's going to hurt you. I don't like either one of them.

INSIGHT STAGE

T1: We need to move on to starting to think about what fits for you [the dreamer] and how you might tie some of this in with what's happening in your life recently.

D: I guess there are several levels. I'm trying to get out of a relationship that's not good for me at all. Although I've never pictured [boyfriend] as a snake, he's dangerous and a lot like my mother, very manipulative and says things as jokes that are cruel. I don't know why it turns into a kitten—that's the one part I can't understand. Then on a generic level, I was thinking that I'm avoiding intimacy, and that if I would just let go and let it happen, it would turn into this kitten. But I obviously still have problems with that demanding part too, not as dangerous, but it's something I'm working on because I have the tendency to be the opposite of dependent. It's like I don't need anything or anybody. I have a tendency to pull away when I do get close to somebody. But the snake could be my mother too. She's driving me crazy now. She's just like that. She's that type of mother that wants to know everything about you. She takes over everything of mine. I can't seem to say something to her without her analyzing this or just taking it over. I feel guilty about saying, "Back off." I kind of created a nightmare for myself because I have my own business with another woman. When you go to conventions we need extra help, so 2 years ago we hired our mothers. They do a great job, and they work very hard. But my last convention was living hell for me to be surrounded by her and working with her for a week. I'm an adult running a 5,000-people convention, and she's trying to tell me what I should wear. This dream could be about that because I'm dreading going down to the next convention. I'm really vulnerable right now.

C5: Is she going to be at this convention?

D: Oh yeah. I'm really scared of how I might react to her because I'm at a point where I'm overreacting. Everything she does now just annoys me.

C3: You feel like she's trying to control you like you were a little girl?

D: Yeah. She's a very controlling person, even though she doesn't see it.

C4: What could you give your mom to turn her into a kitten?

D: The problem is I don't want her to turn into a kitten because she'll be very demanding.

T2: How does she turn into a kitten?

D: Well, through my whole divorce she was very supportive. She can be very nice. My mom is codependent on me. She grew up in a home with a severe alcoholic, and she won't do anything about it. She still calls me a little girl. When she read my diary, she said she had the right to do that because she's my mother. She thinks she owns me. It's my fault now that she's decided that she's going to become a planner. She's attending these seminars and wanting to use my business cards. It's like I've created a monster. But she's trying to take over my life too, now she wants to do what I do, and I don't know how to draw the line.

C4: Can you put up a sign up and give her away?

D: Maybe I want to give her away to my brothers.

T1: It sounds like there's two relationships happening at the same time that make you feel trapped—your mother and your boyfriend.

D: It's the first time I've seen similarities between somebody I'm dating and my mother. I get the same rate of stress that has to do with my mother. He's actually cruel sometimes.

T1: You're powerless with him like with your mother.

D: Yeah.

T2: How is this different from your marriage?

D: My husband was demanding in a different way. He was more like a child—couldn't do anything for himself. He was very successful at his job, but he was incapable of doing anything else. But he never made me feel guilty or anything like that. It was different.

T2: If he was in the dream, what would he be?

D: He definitely wouldn't be the snake. The only thing he could be would be the kitten.

T1: Could the snake and the kittens be different parts of you?

D: I'm not sure.

T1: Is there a part of you that is scared and demanding?

D: I would say, "definitely yes." Because I was raised by my mother, I have a lot of her characteristics that I abhor, but unfortunately I have them. That's what I'm trying to get resolved or get rid of. So yes, I do find sometimes that I can be as manipulative as my mother. I don't like it, but I know I do it.

T1: With yourself or in relationships?

D: Just in relationships. I have a very difficult time saying what I want. I'd rather go round about or write a note or just try to make someone read my mind and figure out what I want. Or I'll find it doesn't matter to me. But whatever matters to me, I'll go out and buy what I want. I'm not good at that, but I'm learning. But I don't know what the snake part would be. I could see the kitten part, but I don't know what snake part would be. I don't feel like it's any part of myself.

T2: Is there a part of yourself like the kitten, a little bit demanding but not as forceful about getting attention?

D: It doesn't feel like that as much as different persons. I could see little spiders being part of myself. I'm not saying it couldn't be. It could very well be, but it's not connecting.

T1: It's an easy translation to think about the snake being the superego part of you, and you are kitten or id or child.

D: The superego would be the snake. Ever since I read about it in psychology, I felt like I had an overdeveloped superego. I definitely have a big voice in my head that's always criticizing me or observing instead of letting me experience.

T2: Is there a part of you that feels as if you were the animal that needs to be given over?

D: I don't think that I want a man to take care of me. Maybe there is some part of me that feels it would be easier that way. To me the easiest thing I could have done was to stay married and not deal with it. Maybe just on the level if I had a man, I could give myself over to him and not deal with anything else, which I know isn't true, but maybe there's that Cinderella thing still around.

T1: Could you each relate how you would interpret this if it were your dream?

C5: I'm very impressed that you're able to hold this thing pretty much at bay and get it to metamorphosize back to a relatively harmless kitten. When we first convened, I had mentioned I had done a little reading about lucid dreaming. There are some cultures where they practice the techniques of not only becoming conscious during a dream but also forcing other images in the dream to change into something else willfully. In one culture in particular, they would do exactly what you just did—make that thing turn into something harmless and demand to give it away. I'm just terribly impressed about the fact that you . . .

D: . . . That I'm making progress. I don't know if my dream is telling me that I'm okay.

C5: It occurred to me that I've had snake dreams before too. I have snake phobia. But if this was my dream, the snake would have gotten to me and probably bitten me right here. I would know at that point that I was going to die within about 3 minutes from a snake bite. There wouldn't have been anything I could do about it before I was able to get it to change back to a kitten. I would have been remorseful that I wasn't able to use my power at that point to get the snake to change to anything else. The snake would win. I don't die in the dream. I just wake up.

C4: If this was my dream, I would have burned myself turning on the hot water. I would have stared down at my feet, would have really hurt. I would have run downstairs and locked that door. The snake would not have headbutted the door, it would have actually burst through the glass and shattered everything. It would not have been this relatively harmless headbutting. It would have been making a huge noise. Probably both of my brothers would have been downstairs, one of whom would have said, "It's not my problem, and I don't know what to tell you. I think maybe what you should do is just run out of the house and hide," because that's what he does emotionally. The other one probably would have gone very much into it and said, "Pay attention to what it wants and give it what it wants and just remain cool and everything will be fine."

D: What you said triggered something in terms of being myself. I want things to work right away. When you try to force things, they don't work out. So I've been trying to just not force things. I have a real hard time with not trying hard. When you said that maybe the snake gets me, and I'm trying to force all these things on myself, and my brother said to let it come near me, I did think of myself as a snake just pushing myself so hard and never getting anywhere. That's what I do. I'm pushing and always analyzing instead of just letting it happen.

T1: There's another part of you that you're not letting be free.

D: I know that if you try to work on something too hard, then once again you're watching yourself trying to make yourself do something instead of letting the process happen. I'm a real impatient person. I want everything to happen right away. I think I want to control it too, just in case something happens that's not the way I like it. I think that's what was happening in the dream. Once it started, I wanted to control it. It took me so long to write it down, because I couldn't connect why my brother would say, "All you have to do is stop and let it come to you and it will." That's what I did, and it turned into a cat. I still wasn't real pleased with the cat.

C3: If this is my dream, I would want the snake to get out of my face and stop trying to control me. Again it gets back to how you have to be everything to everybody. The same thing really with the kitten, I would just look at it and say, "I'm not ready to play right now because I want to do something, and you're just going to have to wait for a little while." I think that would be my dream. I'd say, "Hey, lay back because that's what I'm doing, and when I'm ready, I'll do it." I guess I'm kind of similar to you because I'm impatient and stuff. It's taken me a long time to learn that the impatience makes frustrations. If you want something done quickly, sometimes it's not going to get done quickly and you frustrate yourself even more. I've learned just to try not to push myself. I'm still learning that.

C2: I would rather deal with the snake than the kittens so I would have fought with the snake. I wouldn't have let it turn into kittens. If that was true for me, it would have been either work, which would be my [career], or it would have been a threatening sexual image that I would have been fighting with.

T1: You would have fought it directly, taken it on somehow?

C2: Yeah, I would have fought it in some direct way, and I would have been scared by that. I was scared when she was telling the dream about the snake.

T2: So you see yourself in physical confrontation with it instead of running away from the dream?

C2: I can imagine putting my hands on it, trying to get it away, trying to control it, and kill it.

T2: Do you have sense of whether you would have killed it or whether it would come back?

C2: I don't know. I came from a family that was really crazy. Before [my current career], I made my living as an artist. Both of those are callings, not jobs. They're low-paid, glamorous callings. One of the things that you get out of those is that you belong to a community. A lot of times these bosses have been like fathers. It's interesting, and it's very exciting, and you can do a good job, and they tell you it's good, and you produce this work and live up to things. There are a whole bunch of things about it. It's probably too complex to get into. For me the issues of work would carry along with all these complicated scenarios. Lots of times my bosses were Indian men, so that's why I said it would probably be about work for me.

ACTION STAGE

T2: Let's do action. What can you do differently?

D: I can relax. I can just try not to be so hard on myself. I realize something else. I know I have to get out of this relationship. But the other thing I thought about being so hard and stuff is that when I thought about giving these animals away to a man, well I've been separated for a year. I was doing fairly well, started to feel like I was getting my life back together 6 months ago when I met [boyfriend]. When I got involved with this relationship, I sort of lost the focus on myself. The focus went to the long-distance relationship, to seeing each other every weekend, and talking on the phone. I sort of lost focus about what I was supposed to be working on and improving so that my next relationship wouldn't be the same. I never really finished working on myself. I moved here to get married. I don't have friends in this area, and I never built a life because I got married and lived his life. So I sort of put myself in a predicament where I just gave my life over to a man again. It's almost easier for me to do that than to deal with the actual issues I need to deal with. Now that I realize it, hopefully I'll be able to get out of this relationship, get the courage to do it, start really working on the issues that I need to do. I think I'm ready to do it. But I'm not going to do much this week because the convention is going to take up all of my time. I'm going to just try to go along with the process and not force things because even when I try to visualize, I force things. I am going to think about how to end this thing with [boyfriend]. That's about probably all I'll be able to do this week. I feel like I'm getting closer to getting ready for it. I'm just not there yet.

T2: It sounds like things are going to be very busy for the next couple of weeks, but if you gave yourself 15 minutes a night before you went to bed just to get in tune with yourself and your feelings, are you more likely to err on the side of forcing yourself to feel versus just letting yourself have that 15 minutes to relax and think?

D: I could do it as long as I wasn't in bed. If I was in bed I'd end up either forcing it or falling asleep.

C4: You don't share a room with your mother or anything?

D: No, that would be horrible. One time someone thought she would be nice and put me in the room right down the hall from her. I thought I was going to die. I mean, she's my hired employee. I pay her and she works hard, but I feel guilty the whole time I'm at a convention because I'm not spending time with her or going out to dinner with her. It's not that she's demanding it of me. I just feel terribly guilty, and I hate feeling that way.

T1: Is there any little symbolic thing that you could do that would remind you of your boundaries?

C4: I have a great idea. It sounds to me like you want to keep your relationship with your mom on two different levels. One is as an employee and she does a great job and everything is wonderful there, and another one is that she's your mother and you've got some problems that you're dealing with there. Could you create two boxes and move her picture in the morning from the box that says Mother to the box that says Work? And then just sort of feel like, "Okay, I'm going to deal with this box today?"

D: Well, I don't know how, but I have got to explain to her that she is my employee, and there's some things she just can't do. Like there's this man, a jerk who never leaves me alone, but he's a very important person so I have to be nice to him. Last year he asked me out to dinner. I said, "I'm sorry, thank you, but my father's coming in town," which he was, "and I want to spend time with him." She butts in, "Don't feel obligated by that, you go do what you want, your father's not going to care." I was beyond livid. It put me in a really bad situation. I had to say, "No, I really want to see my father." It was terrible. I haven't forgiven her for that.

T1: You obviously can't fix everything that's wrong between you and your mother before your convention, but is there a little something you could do, even like a token to bring with you to remind you? I can remember a time in my life, I was having a hard time making space for myself in the middle of other relationships. I had a ring that I just loved that I made it to mean that I get to be myself. I wore that ring all the time to remind me that I got to be myself, I got to have my own say, and I could say "No," however I could come up with to say "no" to these other people. I wonder if there's something like that you could take with you or make to remind you that there's more than just these demands put on you by your mother.

C4: If that had been another employee, you would have said to that employee that that was inappropriate.

D: I don't think another employee would have done that.

C4: Okay, but let's assume that another employee did.

D: She jumps the gun. I unfortunately don't have the courage to tell her, except when I go into a rage. I don't seem to be able to sit her down. I tried it a while ago to sit her down and explain. It turned out horrible. She gets so defensive and mean. She cries, and I feel terrible. She says things like I don't love her, I've always been a cold child, and I never let her hug me.

C4: But those are side issues.

D: I know, but she still gets to me. I haven't worked it out enough that I can say anything.

C4: But if you can start from a spot where you can even do a little bit of separation of this is an employee and if another employee had done that, I would have said to them, "That was inappropriate conduct, this is my business, and I was handling that situation in a way that was important for me to handle, your interruption was inappropriate, please do not do that again." You would have said that to another employee.

D: Right, well no, I wouldn't have, but . . .

C4: You would have thought it or wished it. You wouldn't have felt guilty if you had started the conversation, where with your mom you would have. But if there's something symbolic that you could do that reminds you that you employ this woman who happens to be your mother, that that's a different relationship.

T1: Does any little thing comes to mind that you could do, that would remind you that there are some appropriate boundaries there and that your mother stepped over them, to just kind of help remind you to try to shore up your boundaries for the time being?

D: Nothing is popping into my head right now, but I can probably think of something.

T1: If there's something you could take with you or do before you leave or something that would mean something like that for you.

C4: I know some people who would develop a chant like, "I am grown up, I own a business, I am grown up, I own a business."

T2: If you have a belt or a pin or something that you can try to symbolize as this makes me superboss or something that instills that type of thing, something that you can look at and say, "I only wear this when I am doing career stuff, this is my power." Why don't you think about that?

D: Yeah, I'm sure that there's something like that.

T1: Let's go around and have people talk a little bit about their actions. We can come back and see if you've thought of something.

C3: It makes me feel so good after being in another group that was so negative, hearing nothing about empowerment, hearing nothing about visualization, I really feel good.

D: Okay, I know what I'll do. I mean, I don't know if I'll do it, but I think I'll do it. She's always criticized me about the way I've dressed. It's always been, "You're not going to wear that, that's wrinkled." Maybe I'll wear something underneath that like totally clashes with what I have on or something. (*laughter*)

C4: Maybe could you get heels high enough to make you taller than she is. (*laughter*)

D: When your family is tall, heels don't help.

C2: Make her sit somewhere that's drafty, maybe that'll shut her up. She could get laryngitis.

D: The most terrible thing is that she's so proud of me. I hate to make her into a terrible person. It's just that she doesn't know how to be. It's so sad because she wants to have a good relationship and be my friend. I told her she can't have it if she does what she continues to do. She just can't.

C4: It sounds like she's not really happy for you, it sounds like she's sort of . . .

D: Like she's maybe proud of me because she's living her life through me. Yeah, that's true.

T1: We really need to hear how everybody would change if this were their dream.

C4: She was talking about mothers and stuff. I still haven't sat down with my mom and said we need to have this talk. If this were my dream, there would probably be pieces of it that belonged to my relationship with my mom because my mom does that kind of stuff too. I need to go back to the option I didn't take last week and specifically say, "There are things we both need to talk about."

T2: Have you made a list of the things you need to talk to your mother about?

C4: Not, not written down. I do need to do that.

T2: That would be a helpful first step. We need to get on because we're out of time, so if people could be like really concrete about how they would make an action step that would be helpful.

C5: You don't have to worry about me because I'm drawing a total blank out of this whole part of the session. I don't understand how we're supposed to get something out of somebody else's dream.

T2: You said that if this was your dream the snake would have bit you and you would have been dead. So what could you do in your life so that when things are definitely going to strike out and hurt you . . .

C5: I still better pass. I'm not coming up with anything. I'm sorry I can't be more helpful.

T1: Why don't you think about that over the next week and maybe we can touch base with that the next time when we're going back around and give you a little bit more opportunity since you feel a little bit rushed. C2?

C2: I'm trying to sort out personal issues and have them be different from work.

T1: What are you going to do within the next 2 weeks that will help you do that?

C2: Well, I am trying to do two experiments that I think are important and that I like to do rather than ones that someone else wants me to do.

T2: C3?

C3: Today I was struck in close. My ex-husband was totally cursing at me in front of his attorney, and my attorney and I did not feed into his little whim. I sat there looking directly through him. I'm hearing not only my attorney telling him to shut his mouth, but his attorney telling him to shut his mouth. I'm saying, "Oh my God, somebody else is hearing this besides me." It was a different way of me striking out at him because he would never do this in front of other people, to allow people to see what he was like. I don't know how that happened, but it did, and I was very happy about that. Just sitting there and looking directly through him and not acknowledging him or his presence made me feel very good. I could apply it to other people and utilize that same technique. I learned a lot today.

COMMENTARY

This transcript is a wonderful example of how group process works with dream interpretation. By having each person relate to the dream as if it were her own, the dreamer was provided with lots of different ideas to try on about the dream. The group was very involved in trying to help this woman understand her dream. In addition, most of the group members were able to project into the dream and learn a lot for themselves. The energy created by this group working together to understand this woman's dream was very exciting. This woman probably learned more from the group dream interpretation than she would have learned by working on it alone or with an individual therapist.

This dream exemplifies how dreams cannot be interpreted without knowing the individual's personal associations. For example, using Freudian or Jungian symbolic interpretation, one might guess that the snakes were phallic symbols or mesmerizing creatures. Although such symbolism was meaningful for some of the group members, it did not lead to much personal insight for the dreamer. She mentioned that snakes were phallic, but the rest of her associations went in the directions of her current romantic relationship and her relationship with her mother.

The transcript also provides a nice example of how exploration of the dream images leads directly to the underlying conflicts and then flows naturally into a discussion of what the dreamer can do differently in her life on the basis of what she has learned in the dream. The cotherapists gently guided the group by structuring the process but were able to let the group do most of the work in the different stages. The therapists also constructively gave their own associations to some of the images. The therapists were obviously very involved with the dream and the dreamer, but they were also able to stand back and allow the group to work. The cotherapists worked together well, probably because they had a close relationship prior to running the group and felt they could trust each other.

The therapists had to monitor the group closely. Some clients were eager to push their own interpretations onto the dreamer, others wanted the attention themselves, and others withdrew from involvement. Running the group was a balancing act with trying to keep everyone involved and yet keeping the focus on the dreamer. In addition, the therapists needed to keep the dreamer focused because she sometimes went off into extraneous details (most of which are not recorded here), which diverted the attention of the group.

Time was also a crucial issue because the therapists needed to get through all the stages in a relatively short period of time and focus on both the dreamer and all the other group members. In the future, the therapists might want to allow 2½ hours for each group session so that they do not feel so much pressure to rush people through the stages.

In addition, this transcript illustrates how therapists need to be somewhat flexible in using the model. Although they can instruct group members in the stages of the model, group members often go out of sequence. For example, one group member asked about links to waking life before the associations were completed. The dreamer was able to give some preliminary responses, which were interesting, although her responses changed by the time she had associated more completely. In addition, the therapists did not go through the associations in sequence, but they did get to many of the images. Obviously, they could not cover all the images because of time pressures, so they had to select what they believed were the most important images for the associations. If the group had been able to work with this dream longer, they probably would have come up with many more ideas about the meanings of the dream for all the group members.

The therapists did a good job of helping the client come up with an action plan. The whole group provided lots of suggestions for what the dreamer could do differently. The client then picked something that fit best for her—wearing something under her dress that clashed. Although this clearly was not bold enough for some of the other group members or the therapists, it was what the client felt was acceptable personally. As mentioned earlier, the dreamer is always the one who has the ultimate right to decide what the dream means and what she wants to do about it.

Finally, I should comment on the fact that one group member had a hard time projecting onto the dream. She could not go beyond the fact that it was the dreamer's dream and play with it "as if it were her own." Unfortunately, there was not enough time in this session to work with this issue, but therapists would want to talk about such an issue directly with the group and explain the rationale for the projection intervention. It is important to keep the whole group involved in all the stages.

PART IV

❦

Empirical Research
on Dreams and Therapy

CHAPTER TWELVE

A Review of the Research on Dreams and Therapy

ALTHOUGH THOUSANDS of books and articles have been written on dreams and dream interpretation over the centuries, surprisingly few empirical studies have been conducted on the efficacy of dream interpretation. In this chapter I review the few existing studies in the hopes of stimulating more and better research.

The research on dreams and therapy can be divided into the following five areas: (1) the efficacy of dream interpretation, (2) the process of dream interpretation, (3) individual differences in client responsiveness to dream interpretation, (4) the use of dreams as preparation for therapy, and (5) changes in dreams as an index of therapy outcome. The term "dream interpretation" is used generically in this chapter to refer to all methods of working with dreams in therapy.

THE EFFICACY OF DREAM INTERPRETATION

In this section, I consider all studies that examine the outcome of dream interpretation, or change that accrues as a result of dream interpretation. Studies involving both individual and group treatment approaches will be included. Details of the empirical studies are presented in Table 12.1 so that readers can compare methods and results.

Clinical Case Studies

Anecdotal accounts about the importance and efficacy of dream interpretation in therapy have proliferated since the time of Freud, typically from therapists who extol the use of dream interpretation in their

TABLE 12.1. Summaries of Empirical Studies on the Process and Outcome of Individual and Group Dream Interpretation

Study	Clients	Therapists	Design
Cogar & Hill (1992)	67 nondistressed undergraduate volunteers who received course credit	6 doctoral students and 2 PhD therapists; all did readings, had a 2-hour workshop, and had ongoing supervision	Dream interpretation + dream monitoring ($n = 20$) vs. dream monitoring ($n = 24$) vs. control ($n = 23$)
Diemer, Lobell, Vivino, & Hill (1996)	25 adults from the community who volunteered for therapy, were at least moderately distressed, and remembered their dreams	20 doctoral students and 3 experienced therapists; all did readings, had a 6-hour workshop, and had ongoing supervision	Within-subject analysis of dream interpretation sessions vs. event interpretation sessions vs. unstructured sessions ($n = 25$)
Falk & Hill (1995)	34 adult women undergoing recent separation or divorce in treatment	8 doctoral students; all did readings, had a 6-hour workshop, and had ongoing supervision	Dream group ($n = 22$) vs. waiting-list control ($n = 12$); there were 4 groups, each with 4–6 group members and 2 co-leaders
Hill, Diemer, Hes, Hillyer, & Seeman (1993)	60 nondistressed undergraduate volunteers who received course credit	4 doctoral students and 1 experienced therapist; all had at least 1 semester course in dream interpretation, additional practice using model, and ongoing supervision	Own dream vs. another person's dream vs. own troubling event

Measures	Time in therapy	Results	Comments
Pre-, post-, and follow-up on Coopersmith Self-Esteem Inventory and SCL-90-R	6 1-hour individual weekly sessions for dream interpretation condition	No differences between 3 groups on Coopersmith Self-Esteem Inventory or SCL-90-R	Measures not appropriate for well-functioning clients; therapists may not have been trained well enough; 6 sessions may not have been enough
Pre-, post-, and follow-up on SCL-90-R, IIP-S, and insight into dreams and events; pre-therapy on the PSC, PM, and the Openness scale; client and therapist postsession ratings of Depth, WAI, MIS, & SIS-U; process ratings of cognitive complexity in 2nd dream interpretation session	Within the course of 12 sessions of therapy, each client received 2 sessions of dream interpretation, 2 sessions of event interpretation, and 8 unstructured sessions	No differences between types of sessions on postsession measures; none of the measures of psychological mindedness were related to session or treatment outcome; cognitive complexity in dream session was related to session and treatment outcome	Client ratings of depth and understanding were more than 1 standard deviation above norms, which may have caused a ceiling effect; clients were not recruited for having troubling dreams nor did they report dreams spontaneously within therapy
Pre–post on BAI, BDI, Impact of Events Scale, Self-Esteem Scale, insight in dreams; process ratings of involvement and group cohesiveness	8 2-hour group sessions; 1 person presented a dream at each session	Dream interpretation groups > control on self-esteem and insight	Only 4 groups were conducted
Client postsession evaluations on Depth, Mastery–Insight Scale, Positive Emotionality, Negative Emotionality	1 60- to 90-minute individual session	Own dream > other dream or event on depth and insight	Single session may not generalize to ongoing therapy; clients not necessarily motivated for therapy

(cont.)

TABLE 12.1 (*cont.*)

Study	Clients	Therapists	Design
Shuttleworth-Jordan & Saayman (1989)	21 undergraduate volunteers in midrange of anxiety	1 experienced therapist	Shuttleworth-Jordan & Saayman method of group dream interpretation (1 group, $n = 7$) vs. Ullman method of group dream interpretation (1 group, $n = 7$) vs. waiting-list control ($n = 7$)
D. E. Webb & Fagan (1993)	23 undergraduate volunteers who reported having a recurrent dream at least 4 times a month for a year or more; students received course credit for participation	1 experimenter	Psychological kinesiology ($n = 12$) vs. attention control ($n = 14$)

clinical practices. For example, Merrill and Cary (1975) provided case examples of how dream interpretation in brief analytic therapy helped relieve symptoms and reduce acting out for college student clients. Similarly, Levay and Weissberg (1979) described the benefits of using dreams in sex therapy. Bynum (1980, 1993) and Buchholz (1990) wrote about the benefits of sharing dreams in couples and families. Unfortunately, using these case examples as scientific evidence for the efficacy of dream interpretation is problematic given that they rely only on therapist report with no corroborating empirical evidence. Therapists are undoubtedly biased in their estimates of the effects of their interventions. Furthermore, case examples typically include no controls for testing competing hypotheses. The sheer number of such anecdotal reports does, however, suggest that many therapists believe in the efficacy of dream interpretation.

Psychological Kinesiology

Psychological kinesiology was studied as a method of dream interpretation (D. E. Webb & Fagan, 1993). The theory behind this method is

Measures	Time in therapy	Results	Comments
Pre–post on Fear Survey Schedule; client retrospective ratings of tension on a 10-point fear thermometer for different steps of each method	10 90-minute group sessions	Shuttleworth-Jordan & Saayman method > Ullman method on tension and negative reports from therapist and clients	Only 1 therapist conducted 1 group of each type; Ullman method might not have been conducted as competently as other method; no comparison could be made to control group
Frequency of recurrent dreams over 30 days of recording before and after intervention; qualitative data from exit interview	1 45-minute session	Treatment > control in reduction in recurrent dreams; treatment reports more favorable about experience in psychological kinesiology	Only 1 experimenter with unknown training and unknown biases conducted the sessions in both conditions

Note. SCL-90-R = Symptom Checklist-90-R; IIP-S = Inventory of Interpersonal Problems—Short Form; BAI = Beck Anxiety Inventory; BDI = Beck Depression Inventory; PSC = Private Self-Consciousness Scale; PM = Psychological Mindedness Scale; WAI = Working Alliance Inventory; MIS = Mastery–Insight Scale; SIS-U = Session Impact Scale—Understanding Subscale.

that the body is often more aware of a person's reactions than he or she can allow him- or herself to be verbally, so the authors postulated that using this method would circumvent defenses. Therapists first taught clients how to respond "Yes" or "No" by using different muscle responses. After a dreamer presented a dream and revealed his or her feelings and associations, the therapist asked clients to respond "Yes" or "No" muscularly to a series of questions about the meaning of specific dream images. Through this questioning, the therapist developed an interpretation of the dream.

Subjects in the treatment condition met individually with the experimenter for one psychological kinesiology session. In contrast, subjects assigned to the control group met individually with the experimenter for one session to describe their dreams, give associations, and interpret their dreams with the experimenter listening but giving no interpretive feedback. All subjects recorded their dreams for 30 days before and after the session and participated in an exit interview.

The frequency of recurring dreams decreased for individuals in the treatment condition but not for individuals in the control condition. In addition, individuals in the treatment condition reported less concern about their recurring dream, less sleep loss, and fewer awakenings from the recurrent dream than did control subjects. Treatment subjects were also more likely than control subjects to report that their feelings about the dream had changed, that they had learned something about themselves, and that the dream interpretation was helpful.

One major problem with this study is that only one experimenter was used. The training and identity of the experimenter was not made clear, but it is probable that the experimenter was highly committed to proving the efficacy of psychological kinesiology and may have inadvertently treated subjects in the control condition with less enthusiasm than those in the treatment condition. Thus, therapist enthusiasm rather than the specific treatment might have caused the differences between the two groups. The method also requires an incredibly intuitive therapist who can guess the meaning of the dream images without verbal input from the client. Given that the interpretations came from the experimenter's projections, there is no way of knowing if they were accurate or if clients agreed to please the experimenter. The opportunity for too much therapist persuasiveness could be problematic using this approach.

Individual Dream Interpretation

The efficacy of individual dream interpretation in increasing self-esteem and decreasing symptomatology was studied by Cogar and Hill (1992). Undergraduate volunteers were randomly assigned to one of three conditions. In the first condition, participants monitored their dreams (through keeping a dream diary) and participated in 6 weekly sessions of individual dream interpretation with trained therapists using the Hill model. In the second condition, participants monitored their dreams for 6 weeks, thus serving as a control for attention to dreams. The third condition was a waiting list control in which participants received no exposure to dream interpretation or dream monitoring.

Dream interpretation was not significantly better than the other two conditions in terms of changes in symptomatology and self-esteem. In open- ended questions at posttesting about increases in understanding, clients in the dream interpretation condition did, however, report increased self-understanding, suggesting that measures of self-understanding or insight might be included in future studies.

One could construe the results of this study as indicating that dream interpretation was not effective beyond placebo conditions. Before jumping to this conclusion, however, I would note a number of methodological problems with the study: (1) the clients were functioning well and had little to gain from treatment, especially on the measures of pathology that were used in the study; (2) 6 sessions might not have provided enough time for clients to make changes; (3) therapists might not have been trained well enough in the dream interpretation model, which was still in a very preliminary stage of development; (4) it might have been more effective to embed dream interpretation within brief therapy as is done in most clinical practice rather than using dream interpretation as the sole intervention; and (5) the measures did not assess changes that one would expect from this model (e.g., changes in insight and self-understanding or reduction in troubling dreams). Although there were methodological problems with this study, it was a good first step in our program of research because we began to learn what methods and measures to use to investigate dream interpretation.

Efficacy of Dream Groups

The effects of a group dream interpretation approach for women who were recently separated and divorced was investigated by Falk and Hill (1995). Clients were randomly assigned to a group dream interpretation condition or to a waiting-list control. Each client was the focus of attention for one entire group session, with other group members offering associations, interpretations, and actions as if the dream were theirs (as suggested by Ullman & Zimmerman, 1979). This method permitted the dreamer to use whatever aspects of others' insights were helpful without having to feel that someone was telling her what her dream meant. Having each group member provide their own associations, interpretations, and actions also allowed for all group members to gain something for themselves from the focal member's dream interpretation.

Women who participated in the dream interpretation groups gained more self-esteem and insight than did women on the waiting-list control, suggesting the efficacy of dream interpretation groups for women in the divorce transition. The women did not change in levels of symptomatology and anxiety, which, as in Cogar and Hill (1992), we explained by noting that they were functioning well prior to treatment and may not have been able to change much on these measures. Interestingly, we noted in both studies that people who volunteer for dream interpretation studies appear to be relatively mentally healthy. A limitation of this study was the small sample size and correspondingly low power to detect significant effects. In addition, therapists were relatively inexperienced and received only a few hours of training.

Comparison of Dream Interpretation with Other Interventions

Hill, Diemer, Hess, Hillyer, and Seeman (1993) compared dream interpretation to two other therapist interventions. We reasoned that to examine the effectiveness of dream interpretation, one should compare it to similar interventions to rule out competing hypotheses about the key ingredients of dream interpretation.

The first comparison condition was to interpret someone else's dream using the Hill model. This condition was included to control for the effects of projection. Hobson and McCarley (1977) have proposed that dream images come from random bursts in the brainstem during sleep and that the higher brain makes sense out of these haphazard signals by creating dreams. Hence, in dream interpretation we might take this process one step further and create meaning from the dream during our waking life. If this explanation is true and dreams are indeed random, people could project onto another person's dreams as easily as their own and profit from working with the dream.

The second comparison condition was to interpret a recent troubling event using the Hill model. This condition was included to control for the effects of interpretation. In psychotherapy research, interpretation has been found to be one of the most consistently effective therapist techniques (see review by Spiegel & Hill, 1989). The careful process of attending to each element of the dream and trying to understand how the dream fits into the person's life might be beneficial in and of itself. If this is true, then using this systematic method of interpretation with an event from the person's waking life ought to be as effective as interpreting a dream.

Undergraduate volunteers who received course credit for participation were randomly assigned to discuss a recent dream of their own, another person's dream, or a recent troubling event of their own with a therapist for a single session. Results indicated that clients who received dream interpretation rated their sessions as deeper and indicated that they achieved more insight than did clients who participated in the conditions in which they worked on another persons's dream or a recent, troubling personal troubling event. These results suggest that dream interpretation is more effective than other similar techniques and that the effects of dream interpretation cannot be attributed solely to projection or to the interpretation process. Dreams seem to provide a unique stimulus that helps people gain self-understanding.

A limitation of the study was that each client received only one of the three conditions for a single session, which is quite different than typical therapy. Furthermore, clients were undergraduates who received course credit for participating rather than people who were motivated to seek therapy or who were disturbed enough to be similar to clients who seek therapy. Thus, results might not generalize to actual therapy.

Comparison of Dream Interpretation with Other Interventions within Therapy

As a follow-up to the Hill, Diemer, et al. (1993) study, Diemer et al. (1996) studied the effects of dream interpretation compared to event interpretation within the context of brief therapy. Diemer et al. recruited people who wanted individual therapy (rather than dream interpretation) but only selected people as clients who reported that they remembered and were willing to work on dreams and troubling events in therapy. Twenty-five clients received 12 sessions of therapy from trained therapists. Of the eight middle sessions, two were dream interpretation and two were event interpretation. Clients were prompted to bring in either a dream or an event at the end of the previous session.

The results indicated that the overall treatment involving dream interpretation, event interpretation, and unstructured sessions was effective in reducing symptomatology and increasing interpersonal functioning. The test of the primary hypothesis, however, revealed no differences on postsession measures of quality, self-understanding, and insight for dream interpretation, event interpretation, and unstructured middle sessions. Thus, dream interpretation was not more effective than other therapeutic strategies. Given that the client ratings for all sessions on session quality and understanding were more than one standard deviation above the norms, the results must be interpreted in light of the possibility that ceiling effects may have prevented us from finding differences between the different interventions. In effect, it was hard for dream interpretation to be better than therapy that already was above average.

Although initially disappointing, these results about the equivalence of dream and event interpretation make sense in light of the dream interpretation model presented in this book. Essentially, both dream and event interpretation lead back to the related memories and feelings in the schemata, so both should be effective (see Chapter 4). These results are reminiscent of the findings of the equivalence of different treatments in psychotherapy research (Lambert & Bergin, 1994; Luborsky, Singer, & Luborsky, 1975; Smith, Glass, & Miller, 1980). These results suggest that, although dream interpretation might not be the "royal road" to greater self-understanding, it is probably as good a path as any other. Dream interpretation does not have to be superior to other treatments to be considered useful within therapy. It still may be the treatment of choice for some clients at certain moments within therapy, particularly when used by therapists who value dreams and are competent at working with them.

The contradiction between findings of the Diemer et al. (1996) study and the earlier Hill, Diemer, et al. (1993) study is puzzling. However, the two studies did differ in a number of ways. The Diemer et al. sample was older, from the community instead of being college students, more psychologically distressed, and more motivated for therapy. Furthermore, each client in the Diemer et al. study received all three conditions from the same therapist within the context of brief therapy rather than having only one condition in a single session as in the Hill, Diemer, et al. study. Perhaps if clients are to get only one type of intervention, dream interpretation is preferable. However, within the context of good therapy with clients who have not sought treatment for troubling dreams, it does not seem to make a difference if dreams are interpreted instead of events or therapy as usual. As usual, more research is needed to clarify the discrepancies. Also, better measures are needed to assess the specific effects of dream interpretation.

Conclusions and Recommendations

Three empirical studies found evidence for the efficacy of dream interpretation. D. E. Webb and Fagan (1993) found that psychological kinesiology was superior to a control condition. Falk and Hill (1995) found that group dream interpretation was more effective than a waiting-list control for adult women undergoing a separation or divorce transition. Hill, Diemer, et al. (1993) found that dream interpretation was more effective than interpreting another person's dream or a recent event. However, two studies found no effects for dream interpretation. Cogar and Hill (1992) found that individual dream interpretation was not superior to control conditions for well-functioning volunteer student clients. Diemer et al. (1996) found that dream interpretation was not superior to event interpretation or unstructured sessions within the context of ongoing brief therapy. Hence, we cannot draw any firm conclusions about the effectiveness of dream interpretation.

Methodologies varied across studies by method of dream interpretation (one used psychological kinesiology, four used the Hill model), modality (one used dream groups, four used individual interventions), length (two used a single session, one used 6 sessions, one used 8 sessions, one used 2 sessions embedded within 12 sessions of therapy), and experience level of therapists (one was unclear, one had only graduate students, three had a mix of graduate students and experienced therapists). All included control groups of some kind, but only three used controls that involved placebo comparisons (attention or alternate intervention). Only two assessed about therapist beliefs and expectations. Hence, it is not clear if differences in results are due to differences in methodology. More studies are needed using comparable methodologies to facilitate comparisons.

Some recommendations can be made for future research on the efficacy of dream interpretation. First, regarding measures, it seems crucial to select outcome measures that match the functioning level of the clients. If well-functioning clients are studied, then measures that are sensitive to potential changes in healthy functioning rather than pathology need to be used. Furthermore, measures that are sensitive to the effects of dream interpretation (e.g., insight, dream anxiety and experiencing changes in dreams) as opposed to general therapy (e.g., symptomatology, interpersonal functioning) are needed.

A variable that might be influencing the results is the level of therapist training. In the Cogar and Hill (1992), Diemer et al. (1996), and Falk and Hill (1995) studies, most of the therapists were advanced graduate students who had a minimal amount of training (readings, a 1-day workshop, and ongoing group supervision). In the Hill, Diemer, et al. (1993) study, most therapists were graduate students who had completed a semester course in dream interpretation and so were more experienced. Perhaps further training or greater experience levels would produce different results. We need to know more about the type of therapists and type and amount of training required to develop efficacious dream interpretation therapists.

The question of how best to study the effects of dream interpretation and how to isolate its effects from the rest of therapy remains unanswered. For example, in the Diemer et al. study, dream interpretation built upon the rapport already established in therapy, so it is difficult to separate the effects of dream interpretation from the overall effects of therapy. Questions such as these plague all process and outcome research, of course, because separating the effects of one intervention from the whole of therapy is difficult (see Lambert & Hill, 1994).

Future studies might test the efficacy of dream interpretation versus noninterpretation when clients either are very motivated to work on dreams or report troubling dreams spontaneously in therapy. Clients who are motivated to work on dreams, whose dreams are troubling enough for them to seek therapy, or who spontaneously present troubling dreams in therapy might feel particularly discouraged when these dreams are not dealt with in therapy or are not understood or altered. In addition, researchers might study clients who seek therapy for help with their troubling dreams rather than studying clients seeking therapy for other reasons.

An intriguing area for further study is separating out therapist beliefs about the efficacy of dream interpretation from the efficacy of the intervention itself. As noted earlier, many therapists fervently believe in dream interpretation. Frank and Frank (1991) noted that therapist expectations play a major role in the outcome of therapy. Isolating therapist beliefs will be difficult, of course, but it remains an important design issue with which researchers need to struggle. Clearly, perspectives other than just those of therapists have to be included in research designs, especially when therapists are invested in proving the efficacy of the intervention.

I would remind researchers who are interested in investigating dream interpretation that although the empirical study in this area is relatively new, psychotherapy research in general is a very advanced field. General methodological guidelines from research on counseling and psychotherapy apply to studies of dream interpretation (see Heppner, Kivlighan, & Wampold, 1992; Kazdin, 1994; Lambert & Hill, 1994). Researchers particularly need to be aware of the research findings regarding specific therapist interventions in therapy, particularly on therapist interpretation (see reviews by Hill, 1992; Hill & Corbett, 1993; Spiegel & Hill, 1989).

THE PROCESS OF DREAM INTERPRETATION

Whereas outcome refers to the overall effects of treatment, process refers to what goes on during therapy (see Lambert & Hill, 1994). Researchers cab examine what goes on during dream interpretation as well as changes that occur for the person as a result of the dream interpretation. The details of the studies in this section are presented in Table 12.1.

Comparison of the Process of Two Methods of Dream Group Therapy

Shuttleworth-Jordan and Saayman (1989) compared the process of two methods of dream group therapy with a control group. The same therapist led one group of each type; clients were undergraduate volunteers who scored in the midrange of anxiety. The groups were matched for gender, age, and anxiety level, with students being randomly assigned to one of two treatment groups or a control condition. Both groups involved 10 1½-hour weekly sessions with one dream presented per session. Group 1 received the Shuttleworth-Jordan, Saayman, and Faber (1988) method, which involved four steps: relaxation, presentation of dream, amplification (dreamer and group work together to elaborate dream meaning using associations), and closure. Group 2 received Shuttleworth-Jordan and Saayman's version of Ullman's (1979) method, which involved five steps: relaxation, presentation of dream, group members' projections onto the dream, amplification, and closure.

At the end of each session, clients retrospectively completed a 10-point fear thermometer of how much tension they felt at each step of the therapy process. The researchers viewed moderate to high levels of anxiety as the goal of therapy. Results indicated that dreamers and participants in Group 1 increased in tension during the middle steps and then decreased at the closure step. Dreamers and participants in Group 2 stayed constant in tension throughout the process, with the exception that participants dropped in tension during the closure step. In posttherapy interviews, the therapist and clients in Group 1 reported being highly involved, with none experiencing overwhelming tension or loss of control. In contrast, the therapist and clients in Group 2 reported feeling frustrated with the projection step because it felt forced, artificial, and threatening. Thus, the researchers interpreted the data as indicating that Group 1 was superior to Group 2 and that the group projection method was counterproductive for maintaining involvement in the process.

The authors noted that Ullman, in evaluating the study, had reservations about how well the group projection technique had been implemented. I would concur with this reservation given our experience in the Falk and Hill (1995) study. We did not experience the negative results with using the projection technique that Shuttleworth-Jordan and Saayman (1989) emphasized. In fact, therapists and clients really liked the projection method; it seemed to create lots of ideas, facilitated group cohesiveness, and helped clients feel like they were not alone in feelings that they experienced. Perhaps the manner in which the technique is introduced and the way it is used make a difference. From the description given by Shuttleworth-Jordan and Saayman, it sounded as if group members were not allowed to interact with the dreamer during the projection phase. In our groups, interaction did take place and the dreamer was allowed to respond immediately to projections (see Chapter 11 for an example). These discrepancies raise the issue of therapist training when techniques from orientations other than those espoused by the researchers or therapists are used. To provide a fair test, therapists need to be competent and comfortable in implementing the targeted techniques and believe in their efficacy.

Furthermore, this study was seriously flawed by the use of only one therapist for both treatments. Although the authors thought that using the same therapist for both treatments controlled for therapist factors, using the same therapist across conditions raises serious concerns about the equivalency of the therapist's beliefs and behaviors across conditions. The therapist might not have been as competent doing the group projection technique as the other techniques. Furthermore, the therapist might not have believed that the projection method was useful. Robinson, Berman, and Niemeyer (1990) found that researcher and therapist allegiance to a particular approach was a significant confounding variable in comparative psychotherapy outcome research. Furthermore, we do not know if results would generalize to therapists other than this specific therapist. Another problem was the use of only one group for each type of treatment approach, given that results might not replicate across other groups (cf. Bednar & Kaul, 1978). A further concern was the use of a retrospective process measure of fear; the final outcome of sessions may have influenced clients' perceptions of intermediate process within sessions.

The one measure (Fear Survey Schedule) that Shuttleworth-Jordan and Saayman administered to all participants at pre- and posttreatment resulted in significantly different amounts of variability across groups, so they could not compare the two treatment groups to a control condition. Group 2 showed the most variability, indicating that participants varied most in their response to this group. Unfortunately, because the treatments could not be compared to the control, we do not know whether either treatment was efficacious in terms of outcome.

Cognitive Complexity of Client Dialogue

In the Diemer et al. (1996) study discussed above, we tested whether the cognitive complexity of the dialogue of clients during dream interpretation would predict client and therapist perceptions of session process and outcome. Because we had noted that some clients became more involved in sessions, we reasoned that process variables rather than personality variables might be better predictors of client responsiveness to dream interpretation. Because the Hill model requires a heavy emphasis on cognition in doing associations, we thought that cognitive complexity of dialogue might predict perceptions of session process and outcome. Judges rated segments of the dream interpretation sessions on five scales of cognitive complexity (depth, elaborativeness, personal orientation, clarity, and conclusion orientation), which were then combined to form a composite cognitive complexity score. Results indicated that clients whose speech during dream interpretation sessions was judged to be more cognitively complex had "better" sessions (as judged by clients and therapists). These results lend credence to our observation that certain clients become more involved than others in the activity of dream interpretation. Perhaps it suggests that, rather than using pretreatment trait measures to predict responsiveness to dream interpretation, therapists could determine who would profit from dream interpretation by trying it out and seeing whether clients become cognitively involved. Of course, we need to know more about what therapists do to foster cognitive involvement.

Group Member Involvement
and Group Cohesiveness

In the Falk and Hill (1995) dream group study, group members rated group climate after each session, clients and therapists made sociometric ratings of group member involvement, and judges rated the level of cohesion within sessions for each group. None of these process variables were related to treatment outcome. One explanation is that group member involvement and group cohesiveness are not as important in structured groups as in other types of group therapy. Alternatively, the measures of involvement and cohesiveness might not have been adequate. The measures were not psychometrically strong, although they were typical of what is used in group therapy research. Given that these variables seem important clinically, other measures should be tried.

Assimilation of Feelings

Heaton, Hill, Hess, Leota, and Hoffman (1996) are just completing a study about the process of dream interpretation in a 20-session case study of therapy for a client recruited to work on a troubling recurrent dream. Given that recurrent dreams seem to reflect unresolved ongoing problems, our hypothesis is that dream interpretation will help clients assimilate warded-off material and come to understand the recurrent dream more. Thus, we are examining whether and how one client comes to understand more about specific aspects of her schemata through the interpretation of regular and recurrent dreams. In addition, we are investigating the assimilation levels of the three stages of dream interpretation to provide some external validation of the model.

Conclusions and Recommendations

Given the methodological concerns about the Shuttleworth-Jordan and Saayman study and the lack of replication, no conclusions can be drawn about the inclusion of the projection step for dream groups. However, the study provides a good example of a useful methodology for studying the inclusion of different steps of dream interpretation models, especially if several therapists are used who are competent in using all steps.

Group member involvement and group cohesiveness, at least as they were measured, do not seem to be useful constructs for dream interpretation. However, given their relevance in the group therapy literature, further attempts should be made to operationalize these constructs for dream groups.

Cognitive complexity of client dialogue appears to be a promising variable. We need to learn more about whether certain clients are predisposed to be cognitively complex in sessions and what therapists can do to facilitate cognitive complexity. Hopefully, assimilation will also prove to be a useful variable. Other process variables (e.g., depth of experiencing, quality of associations, insight) also need to be investigated.

We need to learn more about what is involved in the client tasks involved in the Exploration, Insight, and Action Stages of the Hill model (and other models). Client reactions to dream interpretation stages could be studied through postsession inquiries (Hill, 1990) or qualitative analyses (see Strauss & Corbin, 1990). Furthermore, task analysis (L. S. Greenberg, 1986, 1991) would be useful to discover the most effective sequences of stages in dream interpretation.

We also need to investigate which therapist techniques are effective in enabling clients to become involved in the tasks of dream interpretation. An interesting study would be to compare the therapeutic process when therapists encourage clients to come to their own interpretations versus when therapists give clients interpretations based on the therapist's understanding of them or when therapists give an interpretation based on a dream dictionary. I postulate that clients would feel that they had gained more and would take more responsibility for their insights when helped to come to their own realizations than when given an interpretation. Alternatively, clients might feel better if therapists offered a tentative interpretation but then let the client expand on it or use it to think of a similar interpretation.

Other therapeutic issues that need to be studied are how to present dream interpretation in treatment and how to integrate dream interpretation into ongoing therapy. We need to study how clients react to being encouraged to bring dreams into therapy or to not having therapists pay attention to the dreams they bring in. Additionally, we need to compare other methods of dream interpretation (e.g., Freudian, Jungian, Gestalt) to the Hill model of interpretation.

Finally, methods need to be developed to assess other process variables unique to dream interpretation. For example, dream interpretation may help clients gain more access to their experiential or intuitive mode of processing as opposed to their rational–analytical mode (see Epstein, 1994). Another possibility is that working with the metaphors or symbolism in dreams may help clients experience their feelings at a deeper level. Given the centrality of these processes for dream interpretation, we need to try to develop measures and methods to investigate them.

INDIVIDUAL DIFFERENCES IN CLIENT RESPONSIVENESS TO DREAM INTERPRETATION

Cogar and Hill (1992) examined whether level of psychological mindedness and the visualizer–verbalizer dimension of cognitive style moderated client responsiveness to dream interpretation. Results indicated that these two variables were not related to changes at outcome.

Despite the fact that Cogar and Hill (1992) found no effects for psychological mindedness in their study, we still thought that it was a likely moderating variable. The theoretical literature suggests that insightful clients respond better to insight-oriented treatments (e.g., Applebaum, 1973). Furthermore, our clinical experience has been that clients who become most involved in dream interpretation seem to be psychologically minded and open to their experiences. Thus, in the Diemer et al. (1996) study, clients completed the Private Self-Consciousness Scale (PSC; Fenigstein, Scheier, & Buss, 1975), the Psychological Mindedness Scale (PM Scale; Conte, Plutchik, Jung, Picard, & Karasu, 1990), and the Openness Scale from the NEO-FFI (Costa & McCrae,

1992) prior to beginning therapy. Results indicated that none of these measures of psychological mindedness were related to session or treatment outcome (with the exception that the PSC was negatively related to therapist ratings of session depth and client insight in the dream interpretation sessions).

In a current study, we (Hill, Diemer, & Heaton 1996) are investigating a number of variables to determine whether we can predict client responsiveness to dream interpretation. We are investigating whether ability to recall dreams, attitudes toward dreams, visual imagery ability, openness, and absorption are predictive of who volunteers for dream interpretation and who benefits from dream interpretation.

Conclusions and Recommendations

The results of the Cogar and Hill (1992) study suggest that the visualizer–verbalizer dimension is not predictive of outcome in dream interpretation. This result is somewhat surprising because there seems to be some consensus that dream recall is related to cognitive style, particularly to such variables as divergent thinking, associative productivity, imagistic ability, and richness of inner life (Cohen, 1974b; Hartmann, Elkin, & Garg, 1991; Tonay, 1993). Perhaps other measures of cognitive style would be more predictive of the process and outcome of dream interpretation.

The results of the Cogar and Hill (1992) and Diemer et al. (1996) studies suggest that psychological mindedness does not predict responsiveness to treatment. Given that there do seem to be dramatic differences in clients' ability to become involved in dream interpretation, we should not give up on trying to develop measures that predict client responsiveness. Perhaps the measures used still were not sensitive to what we mean by psychological mindedness in therapy. A possible alternative measure of psychological mindedness is one used by Cartwright and her colleagues in their project on preparing at-risk clients for therapy (Cartwright, Lloyd, & Wicklund, 1980; Cartwright, Tipton, & Wicklund, 1980; Melstrom & Cartwright, 1983). They obtained an 85% agreement rate between an intake counselor and a researcher on ratings of clients on "degree of access to feelings and inner life." Ratings on this scale accurately predicted which clients dropped out of treatment (Cartwright, Lloyd, & Wicklund, 1980) and were positively related to dream experiencing (Melstrom & Cartwright, 1983).

Alternatively, researchers could investigate other variables that would predict responsiveness to dream interpretation. Perhaps imagistic ability, ability to fantasize, ability to free associate, attitudes toward dreams, and motivation to work on dreams would be more potent predictor variables.

Another thing to consider is that it may not be just client variables

that predict the outcome of dream interpretation. Therapist characteristics might also predict who is more responsive to and effective at
dream interpretation. As with client dream recall, it might be that an
interest in and a positive attitude toward dreams predicts who is
inclined toward using dream interpretation. In addition, therapists
probably vary their style to accommodate clients at different levels of
ability; thus, the process might differ even though the outcome is the
same.

FOCUSING ON DREAMS
AS PREPARATION FOR THERAPY

Among those seeking help from a university counseling center, Cartwright, Tipton, and Wicklund (1980) identified 48 students who were
judged to be mildly to severely disturbed, low in counseling readiness,
unlikely to remain in treatment for the first 10 hours, and not psychologically minded. All participants were given a socialization interview to
prepare them for what to expect from therapy. Sixteen people who did
not want their sleep monitored went directly into treatment. Thirty-two
participants were monitored for 8 nights in a sleep laboratory; they were
wakened during the middle 4 nights during either REM (n = 16) or
NREM (n = 16) sleep and asked to say what was going through their
minds at that moment. In the morning, these participants were asked
to recall what they could of their dreams and to discuss how the dreams
related to each other and to their lives. After participating in this
preparation program, these 32 participants went into insight-oriented
therapy (not focused on dreams).

Results indicated that 5 of 16 (31%) in the REM condition, 7 of 16
(44%) in the NREM condition, and 10 of 16 (62%) in the no-preparation
condition dropped out before completing 10 hours of treatment. Although not statistically significant, the results were in the predicted
direction, suggesting that the preparation program reduced the dropout
rate. It is interesting to note that dream recallers complained that
therapists did not deal with the dreams that they brought in. When they
had been taught about the value of dreams, it undoubtedly felt confus-
ing and perhaps frustrating not to have their dreams focused on in the
subsequent therapy.

All dreams from the laboratory awakenings were scored for their
dream-like qualities. Reports that qualified as dreams were rated high
on a dream-like quality scale. Combining the REM and NREM conditions, results indicated that those who remained in treatment for 10 or
more sessions had significantly more reports that qualified as dreams
(45%) than those who dropped out of treatment (26%). Interestingly, the
group of 16 participants in the REM condition had a low percentage of

REM reports that qualified as dreams (52% compared to a norm of 80% for young adults), suggesting that people who are at risk for premature termination might be infrequent dreamers.

The client's ability to share personal content with the therapist and ability to express affect during sessions was also rated for the first and tenth (or final) therapy hour. Clients who had been in the REM and NREM conditions and who recalled the most dream-like dreams changed the most from the first to last session. Thus, Cartwright et al. concluded that the preparatory program was helpful to clients, although they cautioned that results could have been due to talking with an interested professional rather than because dreams were discussed. In addition, subjects were not randomly assigned to conditions, so the equivalence of groups is suspect.

Cartwright et al. also conducted a pilot study not utilizing the sleep laboratory. Clients who met the same criteria for being poor therapy risks participated in eight daily sessions. Instead of sleeping in the laboratory, they saw a 10-minute videotape of a dream discussion (from the REM condition in the Cartwright, Tipton, & Wicklund, 1980 study). They were asked to look for meanings that were missed by the dreamer and then to work on their own dreams for the remainder of the hour. Five of the eight (62%) stayed in treatment for 10 or more sessions, a rate that was similar to the REM condition in the Cartwright, Tipton, & Wicklund study. Thus, it appears that the sleep laboratory might not be a necessary component of the preparation program, although it would be difficult to use the program with people who could not spontaneously recall dreams without being awakened in the sleep laboratory.

Cartwright and Lamberg (1992) also reported that researchers in Finland used the sleep laboratory to collect dreams with alcoholic patients whose treatment had stalled. Using the sleep laboratory to collect dreams helped to revitalize therapy, making patients more open to exploring their emotional lives. These results open up the intriguing possibility of using dream interventions to deal with therapeutic impasses.

Conclusions and Recommendations

Focusing on dreams appears to be promising as a method of preparing at-risk clients for therapy. Such programs might also be effective for clients who would not be considered at risk but who could profit from learning more about how to disclose appropriately in therapy. Results, however, need to be replicated with larger samples, random assignment to condition, and with proper controls to determine whether talking with an interested professional rather than focusing on dreams is the active ingredient of the change.

CHANGES IN DREAMS AS AN INDEX
OF THERAPY OUTCOME

In this section, I discuss a number of case reports and studies that have examined changes in dreams as a measure of outcome of therapy. Most reports were not of dream interpretation but were of therapy-as-usual. The case reports and empirical studies in this section are covered in less detail because they are not directly related to the topic of the efficacy of dream interpretation. They do however provide ideas of measures that could be useful in assessing changes due to dream interpretation.

Frequency of Recurrent Dreams or Nightmares

A number of reports have indicated reductions in the frequency of recurrent dreams or nightmares after psychoanalytic therapy (e.g., Cavenar & Sullivan, 1978) and behavior rehearsal, systematic desensitization, or implosive therapy (Bishay, 1985; Cavior & Deutsch, 1975; Greer & Silverman, 1967; Haynes & Mooney, 1975; Kellner, Neidhardt, Krakow, & Pathak, 1992; Marks, 1978; Silverman & Greer, 1968). Three studies that included control groups also found significant reductions in frequency of recurrent dreams and nightmares. Celluci and Lawrence (1978) found that seven sessions of systematic desensitization were superior to nightmare discussion groups and a self-monitoring control condition in reducing the number and intensity of nightmares. Miller and DiPilato (1983) found that six sessions of relaxation and desensitization was superior to a control condition in reducing frequency of nightmares. D. E. Webb and Fagan (1993), in the study discussed earlier, found greater reductions in the frequency of recurrent dreams for volunteer subjects receiving a single session of psychological kinesiology than an attention control condition. Belicki (1992) noted, however, that the distress level of nightmares may be more important than the frequency of nightmares, given that she found that some people were not distressed by their nightmares.

Changes in Dream Content or Structure

A number of therapists have provided clinical accounts of changes in dream content that correspond to progress in treatment. For example, Warner (1983) noted that initial themes of self-depreciation and self-destructiveness were replaced with themes of self-gratification and self-satisfaction after successful psychoanalytic treatment. Similarly, Glucksman (1988) described changes in dreams across the course of three psychoanalytic cases reflecting changes in self-concept, defenses, core conflicts, transference reactions, interpersonal relationships, and affective communications. In addition, Warner (1983) reported that patients changed their views of their analysts in their dreams from cold or threatening figures to helpful colleagues after successful psychoanalysis. Bergin (1970) reported a case in which a client spontaneously reported changes in a recurrent dream after desensitization. Prior to therapy, the client had vivid dreams about the conflict situation from which he would awake in a panic. After the second therapy session, he reported that the same dream imagery appeared but that he was able to continue the dream until a satisfactory conclusion. The client then ceased having the dream.

At the end of rational behavior therapy (not focused on dreams), Maultsby and Gram (1974) asked 68 patients about changes in their dreams. Fourteen of 45 (32%) in the excellent improvement group, 8 of 20 (40%) in the moderate improvement group, and 0 of 3 (0%) in the no improvement group reported changes in their dreams.

These reports suggest that therapists from many orientations have noticed changes in dream content for clients after successful therapy. Of course, without empirical evidence, we cannot substantiate whether these changes actually occurred. Furthermore, without appropriate controls, we cannot determine whether changes were due to the intervention or other variables.

Changes in Dreams Due to a Sensitivity Group

Breger, Hunter, and Lane (1971) examined the effects of a sensitivity group on dreams. The dreams of those who participated in a sensitivity group became more unpleasant, portrayed dreamers and others in less successful roles, and had less positive outcomes after therapy. In contrast, the dreams of the control participants changed in a more positive direction over time. No assessment of outcome of the sensitivity group was made, so it is not possible to determine whether the changes in dreams were representative of positive changes in treatment. In fact, descriptions by group members indicate that the group was an intense and stressful experience that was not necessarily facilitative.

Changes in Dream Experiencing and Anxiety Levels

Hendricks and Cartwright (1978) rated the level of experiencing in dreams of 20 students who slept in a sleep laboratory for 3 nights. Ten subjects who reported having been in psychotherapy were rated as having higher levels of dream experiencing than 10 subjects who had not been in psychotherapy. Because retrospective reports of being in psychotherapy were used rather than random assignment to treatment or nontreatment, it was not possible to determine whether psychotherapy led to higher levels of experiencing.

Hendricks and Cartwright also identified a subgroup of students who were judged to have low experiencing levels. These students met individually with an experimenter for four 1-hour sessions, although the content of the sessions is unclear. No changes were found in ratings of dream experiencing. The sample size was extremely small, and the initial ratings of experiencing levels are suspect because they were based on only a 10-minute segment of an interview. The Dream Experiencing Scale, however, does seem promising for future studies.

Melstrom and Cartwright (1983) compared the dreams of four successful and six unsuccessful clients at pre- and posttherapy. The dreams of successful clients were higher in anxiety to start with and tended to increase more in anxiety after treatment than those of unsuccessful clients. In addition, both successful and unsuccessful clients increased in dream experiencing over the course of therapy. Finally, unsuccessful clients were lower in dream-like fantasy to start with, and they increased in dream-like fantasy more over therapy than successful clients. These results are intriguing but need to be replicated with more clients using better indices of outcome. In addition, more evidence is needed about whether heightened anxiety is actually reflects a positive change in treatment.

Changes in Transference

Carlson (1986) used script theory to study six transference dreams (defined as involving the therapist or an obvious surrogate) recorded during and after a 3-year course of psychoanalytic therapy (not focused on dreams) in a single case. She found a significant increase in positive affects, a decrease in negative affects, more effective initiatives by the dreamer, a decrease in shame-ridden isolation, and the growth of a more confident, independent style of functioning. The results are fascinating but questions remain about replicability given the use of a case study and the use of script analysis, a qualitative approach that may prove difficult for other researchers to use reliably. An additional concern is that changes in the transference dreams cannot be related to the process of the therapy because no record was made of the therapy. The client recorded her dreams for her own purposes and made them available to the researcher after completion of the therapy, so the study used a post hoc methodology.

Conclusions and Recommendations

Case reports and three studies involving control groups indicated that the frequency of recurrent dreams and nightmares seems to decrease after therapy. Comparative studies have not been done with different types of therapy so it is not clear if some approaches are more effective than others in reducing recurrent dreams and nightmares. In the future, researchers should test for changes in both frequency and distress level of nightmares and recurrent dreams.

Contradictory evidence has been reported for changes in dream content and structure. Two empirical studies indicated that dreams change in a positive direction as a result of therapy (Carlson, 1986; Melstrom & Cartwright, 1983), one study found a negative change as a result of a sensitivity group (Breger et al., 1971), and one study found no change after 4 hours of contact with an experimenter (Hendricks & Cartwright, 1978). Unfortunately, outcome was measured in only one study and then it was measured using a single-item rating by therapists, who of course are often biased in favor of noticing changes after therapy. In addition, all the studies have used very small sample sizes. Thus, no firm conclusions can be made about the effects of therapy on dream content and structure because of the meager number of empirical studies, small sample sizes, and variations in therapy approaches and methodologies.

The studies in this section do suggest that changes in the frequency of recurrent dreams and nightmares and changes in dream content/structure ought to be included in studies of dream interpretation. Anxiety, dream experiencing, positive and negative affects, and initiative by the dreamer are all measures that could be considered by dream interpretation researchers.

SUMMARY

A great deal of clinical evidence has accumulated from therapists about the efficacy of dream interpretation, but these reports were subject to bias (e.g., therapist expectations and beliefs may have caused the effects rather than the dream interpretation). Only five empirical studies have been done, with three showing positive effects and two showing no effects for dream interpretation. No firm conclusions can be drawn given the diverse methodologies and the contradictory findings.

In terms of process, only three studies have been done (and one is in progress) that investigate the process of dream interpretation. One suggests that projection is not a useful technique in dream groups, although questions can be raised about the therapist competence in doing the projection step. One suggests that client cognitive complexity is a useful process variable. One suggests that group member involvement and group cohesiveness are not related to treatment outcome, although questions could be raised about the adequacy of the measures. Clearly, replications of these findings are needed and much more research needs to be done in the process area.

In terms of client responsiveness to dream interpretation, only two studies have been conducted. Only two traits (psychological mindedness and the visualizer–verbalizer dimension) have been studied and neither were predictive of client responsiveness. Other client and therapist trait and state variables need to be investigated.

Focusing on dreams as preparation for therapy has been investigated in two empirical studies and appears to be promising. Future studies need to include attention controls and random assignment to conditions.

A number of studies have demonstrated that dreams change in frequency, structure, and content as a function of therapy. Interestingly, changes in dreams have not been examined for dream interpretation.

Obviously, we are just in the initial stages of research on dream interpretation. A multitude of questions remains in this underresearched area. I hope that more researchers will begin investigating this area so that we can begin to determine the efficacy of dream interpretation. There are many exciting possibilities for research in dream interpretation. Just as research in sleep and dreaming has become more mainstream in psychology, I hope that research on dream interpretation will become recognized as an important area of psychotherapy research.

A Manual for Self-Guided Dream Interpretation Using the Hill Model of Dream Interpretation

Clara E. Hill,
Kristin J. Heaton,
and David Petersen

T HIS MANUAL is based on a model of dream interpretation developed by Dr. Clara Hill at the University of Maryland. The Hill model of dream interpretation reflects much of what we currently know about dreams—how they are formed and how they can be used to gain greater self-understanding. This model involves three stages. In the first stage, you will explore your dream in detail, paying attention to the thoughts, feelings, images, and memories that you associate with the various elements or images in your dream. In the second stage, you will use what you have learned about yourself and your waking life to gain insight into the dream—to discover what the dream means to you. In the final stage, you will explore several strategies for acting on what you have learned about yourself through the interpretation of your dream. You might use this information about yourself and about your waking life to solve a problem, to work through a troubling life experience, or to change a problematic behavior.

As you work through this manual, it is important to remember that dreams are very personal. The way in which elements are put together to form a dream and the meaning of these individual dream elements are unique to you, the dreamer. For example, picture a bear in your mind. You might picture a teddy bear or Smoky the Bear, while another person might picture a fierce, terrifying grizzly bear. A single dream element has different meanings for different people, therefore any interpretation of the dream must come from the dreamer, because only he or she can know what individual dream elements mean to him or her. Thus, one cannot use a dream dictionary to determine the meaning of a symbol in a dream. From this perspective, there is no right or wrong interpretation of your dream. Your dream is unique to you, and only you can discover a meaning that seems to "fit" for you.

The success and meaningfulness of your interpretation depends on you. If you follow the steps in this manual carefully and thoughtfully, and answer the questions that follow honestly and completely, the interpretation of your dream will probably be rich and meaningful. Most importantly, relax—there are no right or wrong answers to the interpretation of your dream, only more or less meaningful ones.

Begin on the next page.

STEP 1: WRITE YOUR DREAM

In the space provided below write your dream in the present tense—as if it is happening right now. Be sure to use as much detail as you can, including any feelings that come up for you as you write the dream. For example, you might write the following: *I am running through a dark forest. I feel branches ripping at my clothes. I am out of breath and afraid, but I don't know why I am running.*

Your dream:

Continue on another page if you do not have enough space here.

STEP 2: UNDERLINE DREAM ELEMENTS

Now that you have written your dream, it is time to identify important elements in the dream. In this step, underline *up to 14* elements of the dream from Step 1 that are significant for you. The important point here is to underline the elements that stand out for you the most. For instance, the example from Step 1 may look like this:

I am <u>running</u> through a <u>dark forest</u>. I feel <u>branches ripping</u> at my <u>clothes</u>. I am <u>out of breath</u> and <u>afraid</u>, but I <u>do not know why</u> I am running.

In this example, *running, darkness, forest, branches, ripping, clothes, out of breath, afraid,* and *do not know why* were significant for the dreamer, and were thus underlined.

An element is a piece or unit of the dream. It is also sometimes called an image or a symbol. An element can be a thought or a feeling. It can also be a noun, verb, adjective, or phrase.

You do not have to rewrite the dream here, simply go back to the previous page and underline up to 14 dream elements that hold the most significance for you.

As you go through the remaining steps in the manual, you can go back and add or change the elements that you have underlined.

More than 14 elements may be important to you, but you will probably not have time to work with more than 14 in one session. If you are interested, you can go back and work with the other elements at a later time.

STEP 3: PROVIDE MORE DESCRIPTION OF THE DREAM ELEMENTS

In Step 2 you underlined up to 14 dream elements that were significant for you. Now we would like you explore these elements in greater detail. Table A.1, found on the next two pages, has been provided to help you organize this process.

- First, write down each underlined element in the column labeled "Element," moving *sequentially* from the first underlined element in the dream to the last.
- Next, look at the first element (entered into the first row of the "Element" column). Try to recall any additional details that you can about this element as you think about the dream and write these down in the column labeled "Add more details." These additional details might be things such as colors or smells that describe the element more completely.
- After adding more details about this element, write down any feelings or reactions that you experience when you think about this particular element. Write these feelings or reactions in the column labeled "Feelings."
- Repeat this process for each of the elements listed in Table A.1.

Here is an example using the sample dream presented in Step 1:

Element	Additional details	Feelings
1. *Running*	*Running hard but getting nowhere, sweating, smelling clean air*	*Terrified, somewhat dazed*

- Feel free to come back to this step and add more details to your dream elements as you remember more about your dream throughout the process of completing this manual.

TABLE A.1. Details and Feelings

Element	Additional details	Feelings
1.		
2.		
3.		
4.		
5.		
6.		
7.		

TABLE A.1 *(cont.)*

Element	Additional details	Feelings
8.		
9.		
10.		
11.		
12.		
13.		
14.		

STEP 4: ASSOCIATE TO DREAM ELEMENTS

Now that you have described in more detail the underlined elements of your dream, you are ready to explore these elements more completely. We want you to associate to each element because we want to find out what thoughts, feelings, and memories are associated in your mind with each element from your dream. In this step, we would like you to list the *first five* things that come to your mind when you think of each of your underlined elements. Write your associations quickly and try not to censor whatever comes to your mind. Using the dream element *running* from the sample dream, you might ask yourself several questions:

- What is the first thing that comes to your mind when you think of *running*?
- What does *running* remind you of?
- What might *running* represent for you?
- What is *running*?
- How do you feel when you think of *running*?
- Why do you *run*?
- Pretend that you are speaking to someone from another planet who has never heard of *running*. Tell them all about *running*.

Enter your associations to your dream element into the column labeled "Associations" in Table A.2.

Here is an example of associations to the element *running:*

Element	Associations
1. *Running*	*Trying to escape something* *Gym class* *Like walking only more vigorous and rapid* *Chariots of Fire* *Tiring*

TABLE A.2. Associations to Dream Elements

Elements	Associations
1.	
2.	
3.	
4.	
5.	
6.	
7.	

TABLE A.2 *(cont.)*

Elements	Associations
8.	
9.	
10.	
11.	
12.	
13.	
14.	

STEP 5: LINKS TO WAKING LIFE

In this step, you will explore how each of the underlined elements in your dream relates to events in your waking life. Often, events in our daily lives can trigger the appearance of certain elements in our dreams. These waking life events are important to recognize because they can provide clues to the importance and meaning of the dream elements that they trigger. For each element that you entered into Table A.1, you will explore both recent life events as well as memories of past events that may have "triggered" the appearance of a particular element in your dream. Starting with the first element you underlined in your dream, review the details, the feelings, and the associations to the element that you wrote down in Steps 3 and 4. Now think about what might be going on in your present life that in some way resembles the feelings and/or images that come to mind when you think about this element. Enter these recent waking life events into the "Recent triggers" column of Table A.3.

Next, think about past events that come to mind when you think about this particular element. Do the feelings or images that this element brings to mind remind you of anything that you experienced in the past? Enter any related past experiences in the column labeled "Memories."

Here is an example using the sample dream from Step 1:

Element	Recent triggers	Memories
1. *Running*	*I went running yesterday morning and there were low hanging branches along the path that I took.*	*When I was 5 years old, I was chased by a large dog who broke free of his leash. I had to run really hard to get away.*

Appendix

TABLE A.3. Recent Triggers and Memories

Element	Recent triggers	Memories
1.		
2.		
3.		
4.		
5.		
6.		
7.		

TABLE A.3 *(cont.)*

Element	Recent triggers	Memories
8.		
9.		
10.		
11.		
12.		
13.		
14.		

STEP 6: INTERPRETING YOUR DREAM

Now you are ready for the interpretation of your dream. Your dream can be understood on four different levels:

1. The *dream experience* itself
    - Dreams, like waking events, are experiences that have certain effects on us, that carry some meaning for us. Dreams can tell us about our deepest wishes, desires, and fears, about our creativity and our potential. Having experienced this dream, what have you learned about yourself?

2. Recent *waking events*
    - What did you learn about the waking events that triggered your dream?
    - Did you recognize anything in your waking life that was reflected in your dream?
    - What did you learn about yourself in relation to the waking event?

3. *Past experiences*
    - What did you learn about past experiences based on your dream?
    - How did past events in your life influence your dream?
    - How are these past experiences related to each other or to more recent events?

4. *Parts of yourself*
    - Different elements in our dreams sometimes represent different parts of ourselves. We introject (take in or identify with) parts of other people, and we project parts of ourselves onto other people or things. An example of introjection might be to identify with or take on as a part of oneself the competitiveness observed in one's father. You become competitive because it was a part of your father that you really identified with as a child. An example of projection might be to believe that a friend is angry with you when, in fact, she is not. In reality, you are angry, not your friend—you project onto your friend your own anger because you might find it difficult to be angry with someone who is close to you. Thus, we can learn more about ourselves if we think of different elements in the dream as reflections of parts of ourselves. How are the various elements in your dream similar to parts of you?

Here are some questions to think about as you do this step:

- How does your dream reflect your thoughts, feelings, and concerns?
- What is your dream's "message" to you?
- What new insights do you have about yourself, other people, and/or the world based on this dream?

Choose *at least two* of the four levels for interpreting your dream and write your interpretation in the space provided on the next pages.

Here are examples of the four ways of interpreting a dream using the sample dream:

1. Dream experience	In real life I don't run. The experience of running in the dream was pretty neat in a way. I didn't realize I had that much endurance to get through a forest. In a way I felt really strong in the dream. I actually got into the running. Maybe I am more physical than I thought.
2. Recent waking events	I think I'm feeling angry that my boss is trying to hold me back at work just like that branch held me back. I feel like I work real hard, but my boss only gives me small, busy-work projects. I'm afraid that I'm not going to be able to get ahead. I'll be stuck here for the rest of my life.
3. Past experiences	When I was a kid, I was really afraid of forests because I got lost once in a forest. I think that whenever I am feeling anxious now, I feel like I'm in a forest. I feel trapped as I try to run and get out instead of calmly trying to figure out the best solution.
4. Parts of yourself	I think the branches ripping at clothes represent a part of myself, my pride and need for acceptance, that is keeping me from being more open with people about my dreams. The forest represents my darker side—I tend to keep everything in, holding back my emotions and not letting go of my anger.

Interpretation of Your Dream

1. State the level of interpretation that you are using:

_____

2. Write your interpretation in the space provided below. Be as detailed as possible. Weave your feelings, associations, and links to waking life (Steps 3, 4, and 5) into your interpretation and try to make all the pieces of the dream fit.

Continue on another page if you do not have enough space here.

Interpretation of Your Dream

1. State the level of interpretation that you are using:

_____

2. Write your interpretation in the space provided below. Be as detailed as possible. Weave your feelings, associations, and links to waking life (Steps 3, 4, and 5) into your interpretation and try to make all the pieces of the dream fit.

Continue on another page if you do not have enough space here.

STEP 7: PUTTING YOUR
DREAM INTERPRETATION TO WORK

The interpretation of your dream does not end when you discover more about what your dream means to you. The next step—deciding what you are going to do with this new information about yourself and your waking life—is very important. The following questions are designed to help you use this new information in your waking life. You can think about *either* how to change the dream (#1) *or* how to change something in your waking life (#2). Choose one of the following two options and follow the directions provided for that option.

1. If you could change your dream, how would you change it? This is your chance to change your dream in any way you want. Let your creativity guide you—it's your dream and you can do anything you want to with it. (*Note:* If your dream is troubling, you may want to stop the dream while you are actually dreaming it. To do this, you can wake yourself and tell yourself how you want the dream to change. Then you can go back to sleep. Consult Cartwright and Lamberg, 1992, for more information about how to change bad dreams.) In the space below, describe how you would change your dream if you could change any part of it that you wanted:

- Take a moment to think about the changes that you made in your dream. What do you think your choices reveal about you? Write your answer below:

Continue on another page if you do not have enough space here.

2. Sometimes your dream will reveal areas of your life that you wish were different (e.g., take more time out for yourself, improve your study habits, stop smoking). Is there anything that your dream suggests you need to do differently in your life? These do not need to be major life changes, just aspects of your life that you wish were different or that you would like to change in some way, big or small. On the basis of what you learned about yourself from your dream, write down one or two things you would like to do differently in your life in the first column of Table A.4 (located on the following page).

Once you have written down what you would like to do differently in your life, think about how you might actually go about doing these things, or how you might make these changes in your life. Create a plan of action for yourself. Once again, this does not need to be an elaborate plan. Often, it is better to start out with simple, well thought-out plans that are easy to follow and to integrate into your life. You are less likely to get discouraged and to abandon the plan if it is simple. Try to be as clear and as specific as possible in making your action plan. In the second column of Table A.4, write down your plans for making the changes you outlined in the first column.

Here is an example of ways to make use of your interpretation using our sample dream:

Things I would like to change	How I will go about making these changes
1. *Stop procrastinating on my studies.*	1. *Make a daily schedule for myself with specific times to study for each of my classes.* 2. *Find a quiet place with few distractions and go there to study.* 3. *If I follow my schedule and finish my studies each day, reward myself with time to socialize with friends and watch television.* 4. *If I do not follow my schedule or finish my studies, I cannot watch television or socialize that day.*

TABLE A.4. Making Changes in Your Life

Things I would like to change	How I will go about making these changes
1.	1.
	2.
	3.
	4.
2.	1.
	2.
	3.
	4.

STEP 8: CONTINUED WORK ON YOUR DREAM

There are many ways that you can continue working on your dream in the days and weeks to follow. Some people have used the following techniques to continue working on their dreams.

- Go back and spend more time on your dream using this manual (e.g., work on more elements from your dream or on other levels of interpretation).
- Write about the dream in a journal.
- Make up a song or dance about the dream or draw a picture of some part of the dream.
- Seek therapy to explore yourself and your dream further.
- Devise a ritual based on what you have learned from your dream (e.g., placing a twig on a stream or river and letting it float downstream to signify letting go of a relationship that has ended; wear a pin to remind yourself of what you learned in the dream).
- Have another dream and work on it with this approach.

What ideas do you have for continuing to work on your dream? Write down one or two ways in which you might continue your work on this dream.

1.

2.

Congratulations! You have completed all the steps in this manual. We hope that you have a better understanding of your dream, and perhaps even of yourself and your world. Although working through this manual does not qualify you to interpret other people's dreams, we hope that you will use this method to interpret more of your own dreams. If you run into problems, stumbling blocks, or concerns in interpreting your dreams, we would encourage you to seek professional help.

References

Adler, A. (1936). On the interpretation of dreams. *International Journal of Individual Psychology, 2,* 3–16.

Adler, A. (1938). *Social interest: Challenge to mankind.* London: Faber & Faber.

Adler, A. (1958). *What life should mean to you.* New York: Capricorn.

Alberti, R. E., & Emmons, M. L. (1974). *Your perfect right: A guide to assertive behavior.* San Luis Obispo, CA: Impact.

Ansbacher, H. L., & Ansbacher, R. R. (1956). *The individual psychology of Alfred Adler.* New York: Basic Books.

Antrobus, J. S. (1993). Dreaming: Can we do without it? In A. Moffitt, M. Kramer, & R. Hoffman (Eds.), *The functions of dreaming* (pp. 549–558). Albany, NY: SUNY Press.

Antrobus, J. S., Antrobus, J. S., & Fisher, C. (1965). Discrimination of dreaming and nondreaming sleep. *Archives of General Psychiatry, 12,* 395–401.

Applebaum, S. A. (1973). Psychological-mindedness: Word, concept, and essence. *International Journal of Psycho-Analysis, 54,* 35–46.

Aserinsky, E., & Kleitman, N. (1953). Regularly occurring periods of eye motility, and concomitant phenomena, during sleep. *Science, 118,* 273–274.

Aserinsky, E., & Kleitman, N. (1955). Two types of ocular motility in sleep. *Journal of Applied Physiology, 8,* 1–10.

Baekeland, F., Koulack, D., & Lasky, R. (1968). Effects of a stressful presleep experience on electroencelphalograph-recorded sleep. *Psychophysiology, 4,* 436–443.

Barad, M., Altschuler, K., & Goldfarb, A. (1961). A survey of dreams in aged persons. *Archives of General Psychiatry, 4,* 419–424.

Beck, A. T., & Hurvich, M. (1959). Psychological correlates of depression. I. Frequency of "masochistic" dream content in a private practice sample. *Psychosomatic Medicine, 21,* 50–55.

Beck, A. T., & Ward, C. (1961). Dreams of depressed patients: Characteristic themes in manifest content. *Archives of General Psychiatry, 5,* 462–467.

Bednar, R. L., & Kaul, T. J. (1978). Experiential group research: Current perspectives. In S. L. Garfield & A. E. Bergin (Eds.), *Handbook of psychotherapy and behavior change: An empirical analysis* (2nd ed., pp. 769–815). New York: Wiley.

Beebe, J. (1993). A Jungian approach to working with dreams. In G. Delaney (Ed.), *New directions in dream interpretation* (pp. 77–102). Albany, NY: SUNY Press.

Belicki, K. (1992). The relationship of nightmare frequency to nightmare suffering with implications for treatment and research. *Dreaming, 2,* 143–148.

Benjamin, A. (1981). *The helping interview* (3rd ed.). Boston: Houghton Mifflin.

Bergin, A. E. (1970). A note on dream changes following desensitization. *Behavior Therapy, 1,* 546–549.

Biddle, W. E. (1963). Images. *Archives of General Psychiatry, 9,* 464–470.

Bishay, N. (1985). Therapeutic manipulation of nightmares and the manipulation of neuroses. *British Journal of Psychiatry, 146,* 67–70.

Blanck, G. (1966). Some technical implications of ego psychology. *International Journal of Psycho-Analysis, 47,* 6–13.

Bonime, W. (1987). Collaborative dream interpretation. In M. L. Glucksman & S. L. Warner (Eds.), *Dreams in a new perspective: The royal road revisited* (pp. 79–96). New York: Human Sciences Press.

Bordin, E. S. (1979). The generalizability of the psychoanalytic concept of the working alliance. *Psychotherapy: Theory, Research, and Practice, 16,* 252–260.

Bosnak, R. (1988). *A little course in dreams: A basic handbook of Jungian dreamwork.* Boston: Shambhala.

Boss, M. (1958). *The analysis of dreams.* New York: Philosophical Library.

Boss, M. (1963). *Psychoanalysis and daseinsanalysis.* New York: Basic Books.

Boss, M. (1977). *I dreamt last night.* New York: Gardner Press.

Breger, L. (1967). Function of dreams. *Journal of Abnormal Psychology Monographs, 72* (5, Pt. 2, Whole No. 641).

Breger, L. (1969). Dream function: An information processing model. In L. Breger (Ed.), *Clinical–cognitive psychology* (pp. 192–227). Englewood Cliffs, NJ: Prentice-Hall.

Breger, L., Hunter, I., & Lane, R. (1971). The effect of stress on dreams (Monograph 27). *Psychological Issues, 7*(3), 1–214.

Brown, R. J., & Donderi, D. C. (1986). Dream content and self-reported well-being among recurrent dreamers, past recurrent dreamers, and nonrecurrent dreamers. *Journal of Personality and Social Psychology, 50,* 612–623.

Buchholz, M. B. (1990). Using dreams in family therapy. *Journal of Family Therapy, 12,* 387–396.

Burns, D. (1980). *Feeling good.* New York: Penguin Books.

Bynum, E. B. (1980). The use of dreams in family therapy. *Psychotherapy: Theory, Research, and Practice, 17,* 227–231.

Bynum, E. B. (1993). *Families and the interpretation of dreams: Awakening the intimate web.* New York: Harrington Park Press.

Cann, D. R., & Donderi, D. C. (1986). Jungian personality typology and the recall of everyday and archetypal dreams. *Journal of Personality and Social Psychology, 50,* 1021–1030.

Carkhuff, R. R. (1969). *Human and helping relations* (Vols. 1 & 2). New York: Holt, Rinehart & Winston.

Carlson, R. (1986). After analysis: A study of transference dreams following treatment. *Journal of Consulting and Clinical Psychology, 54,* 246–252.

Carrington, P. (1972). Dreams and schizophrenia. *Archives of General Psychiatry, 26,* 343–350.

Cartwright, R. D. (1966). Dream and drug-induced fantasy behavior. *Archives of General Psychiatry, 15,* 7–15.

Cartwright, R. D. (1969). Dreams compared to other forms of fantasy. In M. Kramer (Ed.), *Dream psychology and the new biology of dreaming* (pp. 361–376). Springfield, IL: Charles C. Thomas.

Cartwright, R. D. (1974). The influence of a conscious wish on dreams. *Journal of Abnormal Psychology, 83,* 387–393.

Cartwright, R. D. (1977). *Nightlife.* Englewood Cliffs, NJ: Prentice-Hall.

Cartwright, R. D. (1978). *A primer on sleep and dreaming.* Reading, MA: Addison-Wesley.

Cartwright, R. D. (1979). The nature and function of repetitive dreams: A survey and speculation. *Psychiatry, 42,* 131–137.

Cartwright, R. D. (1986). Affect and dream work from an information-processing POV. *Journal of Mind and Behavior, 7,* 411–427.

Cartwright, R. D. (1990). A network model of dreams. In R. Bootzin, J. Kihlstrom, & D. Schachter (Eds.), *Sleep and cognition* (pp. 179–189). Washington, DC: American Psychological Association.

Cartwright, R. D. (1993). Who needs their dreams? The usefulness of dreams in psychotherapy. *Journal of the American Academy of Psychoanalysis, 21,* 539–547.

Cartwright, R. D., Kasniak, A., Borowitz, G., & Kling, A. (1972). The dreams of homosexual and heterosexual subjects to the same erotic movie. *Psychophysiology, 9,* 117.

Cartwright, R. D., & Lamberg, L. (1992). *Crisis dreaming: Using your dreams to solve your problems.* New York: HarperCollins.

Cartwright, R. D., Lloyd, S., Knight, S., & Trenholme, I. (1984). Broken dreams: A study of the effects of divorce and depression on dream content. *Psychiatry, 47,* 251–259.

Cartwright, R. D., Lloyd, S., & Wicklund, J. (1980). Identifying early dropouts from psychotherapy. *Psychotherapy: Theory, Research, and Practice, 17,* 263–267.

Cartwright, R. D., & Romanek, I. (1978). Repetitive dreams of normal subjects. *Sleep Research, 7,* 174.

Cartwright, R. D., Tipton, L. W., & Wicklund, J. (1980). Focusing on dreams: A preparation program for psychotherapy. *Archives of General Psychiatry, 37,* 275–277.

Cashdan, S. (1988). *Object relations therapy.* New York: Norton.

Caspar, F., Rothenfluh, T., & Segal, Z. (1992). The appeal of connectionism for clinical psychology. *Clinical Psychology Review, 12,* 719–762.

Cavenar, J. O., & Nash, J. L. (1976). The dream as a signal for termination. *Journal of the American Psychoanalytic Association, 24,* 425–436.

Cavenar, J. O., & Sullivan, J. (1978). A recurrent dream as a precipitant. *American Journal of Psychiatry, 135,* 378–379.

Cavior, N., & Deutsch, A. (1975). Systematic desensitization to reduce dream induced anxiety. *Journal of Nervous and Mental Disease, 161,* 433–435.

Celluci, A., & Lawrence, P. (1978). The efficacy of systematic desensitization in reducing nightmares. *Journal of Behavior Therapy and Experimental Psychiatry, 9,* 109–114.

Cogar, M., & Hill, C. E. (1992). Examining the effects of brief individual dream interpretation. *Dreaming, 2,* 239–248.

Cohen, D. B. (1973). Sex role orientation and dream recall. *Journal of Abnormal Psychology, 82,* 246–252.

Cohen, D. B. (1974a). Presleep mood and dream recall. *Journal of Abnormal Psychology, 83,* 45–51.

Cohen, D. B. (1974b). Toward a theory of dream recall. *Psychological Bulletin, 81,* 138–154.

Cohen, D. B., & Wolfe, G. (1973). Dream recall and repression: Evidence for an alternative hypothesis. *Journal of Consulting and Clinical Psychology, 41,* 349–355.

Conte, H. R., Plutchik, R., Jung, B. B., Picard, S., & Karasu, T. B. (1990). Psychological mindedness as a predictor of psychotherapy outcome: A preliminary report. *Comprehensive Psychiatry, 31,* 426–431.

Coolidge, F. L., & Bracken, D. D. (1984). The loss of teeth in dreams: An empirical investigation. *Psychological Reports, 54,* 931–935.

Costa, P. T., Jr., & McCrae, R. R. (1992). *Revised NEO-Personality Inventory (NEO-PI-R) and NEO Five-Factor Inventory (NEO-FFI): Professional manual.* Odessa, FL: Psychological Assessment Resources.

Craig, E., & Walsh, S. J. (1993). The clinical use of dreams. In G. Delaney (Ed.), *New directions in dream interpretation* (pp. 103–154). Albany, NY: SUNY Press.

Crick, F., & Mitchison, G. (1983). The function of dream sleep. *Nature, 304,* 111–114.

Cushway, D., & Sewell, R. (1992). *Counselling with dreams and nightmares.* Newbury Park, CA: Sage.

Delaney, G. (1988). *Living your dreams* (Rev. ed.). San Francisco: Harper & Row.

Delaney, G. (1991). *Breakthrough dreaming.* New York: Bantam Books.

Delaney, G. (1993). The dream interview. In G. Delaney (Ed.), *New directions in dream interpretation* (pp. 195–240). Albany, NY: SUNY Press.

Dement, W. C. (1955). Dream recall and eye movements during sleep in schizophrenics and normals. *Journal of Nervous and Mental Disease, 122,* 263–269.

Dement, W. C., & Kleitman, N. (1957a). The relation of eye movements during sleep to dream activity: An objective method for the study of dreaming. *Journal of Experimental Psychology, 53,* 339–346.

Dement, W. C., & Kleitman, N. (1957b). Cyclic variations in EEG during sleep and their relation to eye movements, body motility and dreaming. *Electroencephalography and Clinical Neurophysiology, 9,* 673–690.

Dement, W. C., & Wolpert, E. A. (1958). The relation of eye movements, body motility, and external stimuli to dream content. *Journal of Experimental Psychology, 55,* 550.

Diemer, R., Lobell, L., Vivino, B., & Hill, C. E. (1996). A comparison of dream interpretation, event interpretation, and unstructured sessions in brief psychotherapy. *Journal of Counseling Psychology, 43,* 99–112.

Domhoff, G. W. (1993). The repetition of dreams and dream elements: A possible clue to the function of dreams. In A. Moffitt, M. Kramer, & R. Hoffman (Eds.), *The functions of dreaming* (pp. 293–320). Albany, NY: SUNY Press.

Egan, G. (1986). *The skilled helper* (3rd ed.). Monterey, CA: Brooks/Cole.

Elliott, R., Shapiro, D. A., Firth-Cozens, J., Stiles, W. B., Hardy, G. E., Llewelyn, S. P., & Margison, F. R. (1994). Comprehensive process analysis of insight events in cognitive–behavioral and psychodynamic–interpersonal psychotherapies. *Journal of Counseling Psychology, 41,* 441–463.

Enright, J. (1970). An introduction to Gestalt techniques. In J. Fagan & I. L. Shepherd (Eds.), *Gestalt therapy now* (pp. 107–124). New York: Harper & Row.

Epstein, S. (1994). Integration of the cognitive and psychodynamic unconscious. *American Psychologist, 49,* 709–724.

Erikson, E. (1954). The dream specimen of psychoanalysis. In R. Knight & C. Friedman (Eds.), *Psychoanalytic psychiatry and psychology* (pp. 131–170). New York: International Universities Press.

Evans, C. (1983). *Landscapes of the night: How and why we dream.* New York: Viking.

Falk, D. R., & Hill, C. E. (1995). The effectiveness of dream interpretation groups for women in a divorce transition. *Dreaming, 5,* 29–42.

Faraday, A. (1972). *Dream power.* New York: Coward, McCann & Geoghegan.

Faraday, A. (1974). *The dream game.* New York: Harper & Row.

Fenigstein, A., Scheier, M. F., & Buss, A. H. (1975). Public and private self-consciousness: Assessment and theory. *Journal of Consulting and Clinical Psychology, 43,* 522–527.

Field, S. D., Barkham, M., Shapiro, D. A., & Stiles, W. B. (1994). Assessment of assimilation in psychotherapy: A quantitative case study of problematic experiences with a significant other. *Journal of Counseling Psychology, 41,* 397–406.

Fisch, R., Weakland, J. H., & Segal, L. (1982). *The tactics of change: Doing therapy briefly.* San Francisco: Jossey-Bass.

Flowers, L. (1993). The dream interview method in a private outpatient psychotherapy practice. In G. Delaney (Ed.), *New directions in dream interpretation* (pp. 241–288). Albany, NY: SUNY Press.

Fosshage, J. L. (1983). The psychoanalytic function of dreams: A revised psychoanalytic perspective. *Psychoanalysis and Contemporary Thought, 6,* 641–669.

Fosshage, J. L. (1987). New vistas in dream interpretation. In M. L. Glucksman & S. L. Warner (Eds.), *Dreams in a new perspective: The royal road revisited* (pp. 23–44). New York: Human Sciences Press.

Foulkes, D. (1964). Theories of dream formation and recent studies of sleep consciousness. *Psychological Bulletin, 62,* 236–247.

Foulkes, D. (1985a). *Children's dreams: Longitudinal studies.* New York: Wiley.

Foulkes, D. (1985b). *Dreaming: A cognitive-psychological analysis.* Hillsdale, NJ: Erlbaum.

Foulkes, D., Hollifield, M., Sullivan, B., Bradley, L., & Terry, R. (1990). REM dreaming and cognitive skills at ages 5–8: A cross-sectional study. *International Journal of Behavior Development, 13,* 447–465.

Foulkes, D., & Vogel, G. (1965). Mental activity at sleep onset. *Journal of Abnormal Psychology, 70,* 231–243.

Fox, R., Kramer, M., Baldridge, B., Whitman, R., & Ornstein, P. (1968). The experimenter variable in dream research. *Diseases of the Nervous System, 29,* 698–701.

Frank, J. D., & Frank, J. B. (1991). *Persuasion and healing: A comparative study of psychotherapy.* Baltimore: Johns Hopkins University Press.

Freud, S. (1966). *The interpretation of dreams.* New York: Avon. (Original work published 1900)

Freud, S. (1953). Remembering, repeating, and working through. In J. Strachey (Ed. and Trans.), *The standard edition of the complete psychological works of Sigmund Freud* (Vol. 12, pp. 147–156). London: Hogarth Press. (Original work published 1914)

Fromm-Reichmann, F. (1950). *Principles of intensive psychotherapy.* Chicago: University of Chicago Press.

Gackenbach, J., & Bosveld, J. (1989). *Control your dreams.* New York: Harper & Row.

Garfield, P. (1974). *Creative dreaming.* New York: Ballantine.

Garfield, P. (1991). *Women's bodies, women's dreams.* New York: Holt, Rinehart & Winston.

Garma, A. (1987). Freudian approach. In J. L. Fosshage & C. A. Loew (Eds.), *Dream interpretation: A comparative study* (pp. 16–51). New York: PMA.

Gelso, C. J., & Carter, J. A. (1985). The relationship in counseling and psychotherapy: Components, consequences, and theoretical antecedents. *Counseling Psychologist, 13,* 155–244.

Gelso, C. J., & Carter, J. A. (1994). Components of the psychotherapy relationship: Their interaction and unfolding during treatment. *Journal of Counseling Psychology, 41,* 296–306.

Gendlin, E. (1986). *Let your body interpret your dream.* Wilmette, IL: Chiron.

Glass, A. L., & Holyoak, L. J. (1986). *Cognition* (2nd ed.). New York: Random House.

Globus, G. C. (1993). Connectionism and sleep. In A. Moffitt, M. Kramer, & R. Hoffman (Eds.), *The functions of dreaming* (pp. 119–138). Albany, NY: SUNY Press.

Glucksman, M. L. (1988). The use of successive dreams to facilitate and document change during treatment. *Journal of the American Academy of Psychoanalysis, 16,* 47–69.

Glucksman, M. L., & Warner, S. L. (Eds.). (1987). *Dreams in a new perspective: The royal road revisited.* New York: Human Sciences Press.

Gold, L. (1959). Adler's theory of dreams: A holistic approach to interpretation. In B. B. Wolman (Ed.), *Handbook of dreams: Research, theories, and applications* (pp. 319–341). New York: Van Nostrand Reinhold.

Goldfried, M. R., & Davison, G. C. (1994). *Clinical behavior therapy.* New York: Wiley.

Goldhirsh, M. L. (1961). Manifest content of dreams of convicted sex offenders. *Journal of Abnormal Social Psychology, 63,* 643–645.

Goodenough, D. R. (1978). Dream recall: History and current status of the field. In A. Arkin, J. Antrobus, & S. Ellman (Eds.), *The mind in sleep: Psychology and psychophysiology* (pp. 113–140). New York: Erlbaum.

Goodenough, D. R., Witkin, H. A., Koulack, D., & Cohen, H. (1975). The effects of stress films on dream affect and on respiration and eye-movement activity during rapid-eye-movement sleep. *Psychophysiology, 12,* 313–320.

Greenberg, L. S. (1986). Change process research. *Journal of Consulting and Clinical Psychology, 54,* 4–9.

Greenberg, L. S. (1991). Research on the process of change. *Psychotherapy Research, 1,* 3–16.

Greenberg, L. S., & Dompierre, L. (1981). Specific effects of Gestalt two-chair dialogue on intrapsychic conflict in counseling. *Journal of Counseling Psychology, 28,* 288–294.

Greenberg, L. S., & Higgins, H. (1980). Effects of two-chair dialogue and focusing on conflict resolution. *Journal of Counseling Psychology, 27,* 221–225.

Greenberg, L. S., Rice, L. N., & Elliott, R. (1993). *Facilitating emotional change.* New York: Guilford Press.

Greenberg, L. S., & Safran, J. D. (1987). *Emotion in psychotherapy.* New York: Guilford Press.

Greenberg, R. (1987). The dream problem and problems in dreams. In M. L. Glucksman & S. L. Warner (Eds.), *Dreams in a new perspective: The royal road revisited* (pp. 45–57). New York: Human Sciences Press.

Greenberg, R., & Pearlman, C. (1993). An integrated approach to dream theory: Contributions from sleep research and clinical practice. In A. Moffitt, M. Kramer, & R. Hoffmann (Eds.), *The functions of dreaming* (pp. 363–380). Albany, NY: SUNY Press.

Greenson, R. R. (1967). *The technique and practice of psychoanalysis* (Vol. 1). Madison, CT: International Universities Press.

Greer, J. H., & Silverman, I. (1967). Treatment of a recurrent nightmare by behavior modification procedures: A case study. *Journal of Abnormal Psychology, 72,* 188–190.

Griffith, R., Miyago, O., & Tago, A. (1958). The universality of typical dreams: Japanese vs. Americans. *American Anthropologist, 60,* 1173–1179.

Gross, M. M., Goodenough, D., Tobin, M., Halpert, E., Lepore, D., Perlstein, A., Sirota, M., Dibianco, J., Fuller, R., & Kishner, I. (1966). Sleep disturbances and hallucinations in the acute alcohol psychosis. *Journal of Nervous and Mental Disease, 142,* 493–514.

Guntrip, H. (1969). *Schizoid phenomena, object relations, and the self.* New York: International Universities Press.

Gurman, A. S. (1977). The patient's perception of the therapeutic relationship. In A. S. Gurman and A. M. Razin (Eds.), *Effective psychotherapy: A handbook of research* (pp. 503–543). Elmsford, NY: Pergamon Press.

Haley, J. (1973). *Uncommon therapy: The psychiatric techniques of Milton H. Erickson, M.D.* New York: Norton.

Hall, C. S. (1947). Diagnosing personality by the analysis of dreams. *Journal of Personality and Social Psychology, 42,* 68–79.

Hall, C. S. (1953). *The meaning of dreams.* New York: Harper & Brothers.

Hall, C. S. (1955). The significance of the dream of being attacked. *Journal of Personality, 24,* 164–180.

Hall, C. S., & Nordby, V. J. (1972). *The individual and his dreams.* New York: New American Library.

Hall, C. S., & Van de Castle, R. L. (1966). *The content analysis of dreams.* New York: Appleton-Century-Crofts.

Harris, I. (1948). Observations concerning typical anxiety dreams. *Psychiatry, 11,* 301–309.

Hartmann, E. (1984). *The nightmare.* New York: Basic Books.

Hartmann, E., Elkin, R., & Garg, M. (1991). Personality and dreaming: The dreams of people with very thick or very thin boundaries. *Dreaming, 1,* 311–324.

Haynes, S., & Mooney, D. (1975). Nightmares: Etiological, theoretical, and behavioral considerations. *Psychological Records, 25,* 225–236.

Heaton, K. J., Hill, C. E., Hess, S., Leota, C., & Hoffman, M. A. (1996). *Using the assimilation model with recurrent dreams in psychotherapy.* Manuscript in preparation.

Hendricks, M., & Cartwright, R. D. (1978). Experiencing levels in dreams: An individual difference variable. *Psychotherapy: Theory, Research, and Practice, 15,* 292–298.

Heppner, P. P., Kivlighan, D. M., & Wampold, B. E. (1992). *Research designs in counseling.* Pacific Grove, CA: Brooks/Cole.

Herman, J., Roffwarg, H., & Tauber, E. S. (1968). Color and other perceptual qualities of REM and NREM dreams. *Psychophysiology, 5,* 223.

Hersh, J. B., & Taub-Bynum, E. B. (1985). The use of dreams in brief therapy. *Psychotherapy, 22,* 248–255.

Hill, A. B. (1974). Personality correlates of dream recall. *Journal of Consulting and Clinical Psychology, 42,* 766–773.

Hill, C. E. (1985). *Manual for Counselor Verbal Response Modes Category Systems* (Rev. ed.). Unpublished manuscript, University of Maryland at College Park.

Hill, C. E. (1989). *Therapist techniques and client outcomes: Eight cases of brief psychotherapy.* Newbury Park, CA: Sage.

Hill, C. E. (1990). A review of exploratory in-session process research. *Journal of Consulting and Clinical Psychology, 58,* 288–294.

Hill, C. E. (1992). Research on therapist techniques in brief individual therapy: Implications for practitioners. *Counseling Psychologist, 20,* 689–711.

Hill, C. E. (1996). Dreams and therapy. *Psychotherapy Research, 6,* 1–15.

Hill, C. E., & Corbett, M. M. (1993). A perspective on the history of process and outcome research in counseling psychology. *Journal of Counseling Psychology, 40,* 3–28.

Hill, C. E., Diemer, R., Heaton, K. J. (1996). *Correlates of dream recall, volunteering for dream interpretation, and responsiveness to dream interpretation.* Manuscript in preparation.

Hill, C. E., Diemer, R., Hess, S., Hillyer, A., & Seeman, R. (1993). Are the effects of dream interpretation on session quality, insight, and emotions due to the dream itself, to projection, or to the interpretation process? *Dreaming, 3,* 211–222.

Hill, C. E., Helms, J. E., Tichenor, V., Spiegel, S. B., O'Grady, K. E., & Perry, E. S. (1988). Effects of therapist response modes in brief psychotherapy. *Journal of Counseling Psychology, 35,* 222–233.

Hill, C. E., Mahalik, J. R., & Thompson, B. J. (1989). Therapist self-disclosure. *Psychotherapy, 26,* 290–295.

Hill, C. E., & Regan, A. (1991). Therapist use of metaphors in a case of brief psychotherapy. *Journal of Integrative and Eclectic Psychotherapy, 10,* 56–67.

Hill, C. E., Thompson, B. J., Cogar, M. M., & Denman, D. W., III. (1993). Beneath the surface of long-term therapy: Client and therapist report of their own and each other's covert processes. *Journal of Counseling Psychology, 40,* 278–288.

Hill, C. E., Thompson, B. J., & Corbett, M. M. (1992). The impact of therapist ability to perceive displayed and hidden client reactions on immediate outcome in first sessions of brief therapy. *Psychotherapy Research, 2,* 143–155.

Hobson, J. A. (1988). *The dreaming brain.* New York: Basic Books.

Hobson, J. A., Hoffman, S. A., Helfand, R., & Kostner, D. (1987). Dream bizarreness and the activation–synthesis hypothesis. *Human Neurobiology, 6,* 157–164.

Hobson, J. A., & McCarley, R. W. (1977). The brain as a dream state generator: An activation–synthesis hypothesis of the dream process. *American Journal of Psychiatry, 134,* 1335–1348.

Horvath, A. O. (1995). The therapeutic relationship: From transference to alliance. *In Session: Psychotherapy in Practice, 1,* 7–18.

Horvath, A. O., & Symonds, B. D. (1991). Relation between working alliance and outcome in psychotherapy: A meta-analysis. *Journal of Counseling Psychology, 38,* 139–149.

Howard, G. S. (1991). Culture tales: A narrative approach to thinking, cross-cultural psychology, and psychotherapy. *American Psychologist, 46,* 187–197.

Howard, G. S. (1992). Behold our creation! What counseling psychology has become and might yet become. *Journal of Counseling Psychology, 39,* 419–442.

Hunt, H. (1986). Some relations between the cognitive psychology of dreams and dream phenomenology. *Journal of Mind and Behavior, 7,* 213–228.

Hunt, H. (1989). *The multiplicity of dreams: Memory, imagination, and consciousness.* New Haven, CT: Yale University Press.

Ivey, A. E. (1995). *Intentional interviewing and counseling: Facilitating client development* (3rd ed.). Pacific Grove, CA: Brooks/Cole.

Johnson, R. (1986). *Inner work.* San Francisco: Harper & Row.

Jones, R. M. (1970). *The new psychology of dreaming.* New York: Grune & Stratton.

Jung, C. G. (Ed.). (1964). *Man and his symbols.* New York: Dell.

Jung, C. G. (1974). *Dreams* (R. F. C. Hull, Trans.). Princeton, NJ: Princeton University Press.

Kales, A., Malstrom, E. J., Kee, H. K., Kales, J. D., & Tan, T. L. (1969). Effects of hypnotics of sleep patterns, dreaming, and mood state: Laboratory and home studies. *Biological Psychiatry, 1,* 235–241.

Kant, O. (1942). Dreams of schizophrenic patients. *Journal of Nervous and Mental Disease, 95,* 335–347.

Kazdin, A. E. (1994). Methodology, design, and evaluation in psychotherapy research. In A. E. Bergin & S. L. Garfield (Eds.), *Handbook of psychotherapy and behavior change: An empirical analysis* (4th ed., pp. 19–71). New York: Wiley.

Kellner, R., Neidhardt, J., Krakow, B., & Pathak, D. (1992). Changes in chronic nightmares after one session of desensitization or rehearsal instructions. *American Journal of Psychiatry, 149,* 659–663.

Kelly, G. (1955). *The psychology of personal constructs* (Vols. 1 & 2). New York: Norton.

Kiesler, D. J. (1988). *Therapeutic metacommunication: Therapist impact disclosure as feedback in psychotherapy.* Palo Alto, CA: Consulting Psychologists Press.

Kilborne, B. (1990). Ancient and native peoples' dreams. In S. Krippner (Ed.), *Dreamtime and dreamwork: Decoding the language of the night* (pp. 194–203). Los Angeles: Tarcher.

Kleitman, N. (1963). *Sleep and wakefulness* (2nd ed.). Chicago: University of Chicago Press.

Koulack, D. (1991). *To catch a dream: Explorations of dreaming.* Albany, NY: SUNY Press.

Koulack, D., & Goodenough, D. R. (1976). Dream recall and dream recall failure: An arousal–retrieval model. *Psychological Bulletin, 93,* 975–984.

Kramer, M. (1982). Psychology of the dream: Art or science? *Psychiatric Journal of the University of Ottawa, 7,* 87–100.

Kramer, M. (1992). Mood change from night to morning. *Sleep Research, 21,* 153.

Kramer, M. (1993). Dream translation: An approach to understanding dreams. In G. Delaney (Ed.), *New directions in dream interpretation* (pp. 155–194). Albany, NY: SUNY Press.

Kramer, M., Hlasny, R., Jacobs, G., & Roth, T. (1976). Do dreams have meaning? An empirical inquiry. *American Journal of Psychiatry, 133,* 778–781.

Kramer, M., Moshiri, A., & Scharf, M. (1982). The organization of mental content in and between the waking and dream state. *Sleep Research, 1,* 106.

Kramer, M., & Roth, T. (1979). Dreams in psychopathology. In B. Wolman (Ed.), *Handbook of dreams.* New York: Van Nostrand Reinhold.

Kramer, M., Schoen, L., & Kinney, L. (1987). Nightmares in Vietnam veterans. *Journal of the American Academy of Psychoanalysis, 127,* 1350–1356.

Kramer, M., Whitman, R., Baldridge, B., & Lansky, L. (1966). Dreaming in the depressed. *Canadian Psychiatric Association Journal, 11,* 178–192.

Kramer, M., Whitman, R., Baldridge, B., & Ornstein, P. (1970). Dream content in male schizophrenic patients. *Diseases of the Nervous System, 31,* 51–58.

Kramer, M., Winget, C., & Whitman, R. (1971). A city dreams: A survey approach to normative dream content. *American Journal of Psychiatry, 127,* 1350–1356.

Krippner, S. (Ed.) (1990a). *Dreamtime and dreamwork: Decoding the language of the night.* Los Angeles: Tarcher.

Krippner, S. (1990b). Introduction to dreams in different times and places section. In S. Krippner (Ed.), *Dreamtime and dreamwork: Decoding the language of the night* (pp. 171–174). Los Angeles: Tarcher.

Krippner, S. (1990c). Tribal shamans and their travels into dreamtime. In S. Krippner (Ed.), *Dreamtime and dreamwork: Decoding the language of the night* (pp. 185–193). Los Angeles: Tarcher.

LaBerge, S. (1985). *Lucid dreaming.* New York: Ballantine.

Lakoff, G. (1993). How metaphor structures dreams: The theory of conceptual metaphor applied to dream analysis. *Dreaming, 3,* 77–98.

Lambert, M. J., & Bergin, A. E. (1994). The effectiveness of psychotherapy. In A. E. Bergin & S. L. Garfield (Eds.), *Handbook of psychotherapy and behavior change: An empirical analysis* (4th ed., pp. 143–189). New York: Wiley.

Lambert, M. J., & Hill, C. E. (1994). Assessing psychotherapy outcomes and processes. In A. E. Bergin & S. L. Garfield (Eds.), *Handbook of psychotherapy and behavior change: An empirical analysis* (4th ed., pp. 72–113). New York: Wiley.

Langs, R. J. (1966). Manifest dreams from three clinical groups. *Archives of General Psychiatry, 14,* 634–643.

Levay, A. N., & Weissberg, J. (1979). The role of dreams in sex therapy. *Journal of Sex and Marital Therapy, 5,* 334–339.

LeVine, R. (1966). *Dreams and deeds: Achievement motivation in Nigeria.* Chicago: University of Chicago Press.

Levy, S. R. (1984). *Principles of interpretation.* New York: Jason Aronson.

Lewis, H., Goodenough, D., Shapiro, A., & Sleser, I. (1966). Individual differences in dream recall. *Journal of Abnormal Psychology, 71,* 52–59.

Liebert, R. M., & Spiegler, M. D. (1987). *Personality: Strategies and issues.* Chicago: Dorsey.

Loftus, E. (1988). *Memory.* New York: Ardsley House.

Lortie-Lussier, M., Schwab, C., & De Koninck, J. (1985). Working mothers versus homemakers: Do dreams reflect the changing roles of women? *Sex Roles, 12,* 1009–1021.

Luborsky, L., Singer, B., & Luborsky, L. (1975). Comparative studies of psychotherapies: Is it true that "everyone has won and all must have prizes"? *Archives of General Psychiatry, 32,* 995–1008.

Mahoney, M. J. (1991). *Human change processes: The scientific foundations of psychotherapy.* New York: Basic Books.

Mahrer, A. R. (1990). *Dream work in psychotherapy and self-change.* New York: Norton.

Marks, I. (1978). Rehearsal relief of a nightmare. *British Journal of Psychiatry, 133,* 461–465.

Maultsby, M. C., Jr., & Gram, J. M. (1974). Dream changes following successful rational behavior therapy. *Rational Living, 9,* 30–33.

McCarley, R. W., & Hobson, J. A. (1977). The neurobiological origins of the psychoanalytic dream theory. *American Journal of Psychiatry, 134,* 1211–1221.

McCarley, R. W., & Hoffman, E. (1981). REM sleep dreams and the activation-synthesis hypothesis. *American Journal of Psychiatry, 138,* 904–912.

McMullen, L. M. (1995). Methods and metaphors: The study of figurative language in psychotherapy. In L. T. Hoshmand & J. Martin (Eds.), *Research as praxis* (pp. 153–170). New York: Teachers College Press.

Medin, D. L., & Ross, B. H. (1992). *Cognitive psychology.* New York: Harcourt Brace Jovanovich.

Meier, C., Ruell, H., Ziegler, A., & Hall, C. (1968). Forgetting dreams in the lab. *Perceptual and Motor Skills, 26,* 551–557.

Melstrom, M. A., & Cartwright, R. D. (1983). Effects of successful vs. unsuccessful psychotherapy outcome on some dream dimensions. *Psychiatry, 46,* 51–65.

Merrill, S., & Cary, G. L. (1975). Dream analysis in brief psychotherapy. *American Journal of Psychotherapy, 29,* 185–192.

Miller, W., & DiPilato, M. (1983). Treatment of nightmares via relaxation and desensitization: A controlled evaluation. *Journal of Consulting and Clinical Psychology, 51,* 870–877.

Monroe, L. J., Rechtschaffen, A., Foulkes, D., & Jensen, J. (1965). Discriminability of REM and NREM reports. *Journal of Personality and Social Psychology, 2,* 456–460.

Natterson, J. M. (1980). The dream in group psychotherapy. In J. M. Natterson (Ed.), *The dream in clinical practice* (pp. 434–443). New York: Jason Aronson.

Natterson, J. M. (1993). Dreams: The gateway to consciousness. In G. Delaney (Ed.), *New directions in dream interpretation* (pp. 41–76). Albany, NY: SUNY Press.

Noble, D. (1951). A study of dreams in schizophrenia and allied states. *American Journal of Psychiatry, 107,* 612–616.

Olson, H. A. (1979). *Early recollections: Their use in diagnosis and psychotherapy.* Springfield, IL: Charles C. Thomas.

Orlinsky, D. E., Grawe, K., & Parks, B. K. (1994). Process and outcome of psychotherapy—Noch Einmal. In A. E. Bergin & S. L. Garfield (Eds.), *Handbook of psychotherapy and behavior change: An empirical analysis* (4th ed., pp. 270–376). New York: Wiley.

Orlinsky, D. E., & Howard, K. I. (1986). Process and outcome of psychotherapy. In S. L. Garfield & A. E. Bergin (Eds.), *Handbook of psychotherapy and behavior change: An empirical analysis* (3rd ed., pp. 311–384). New York: Wiley.

Palombo, S. R. (1978). *Dreaming and memory.* New York: Basic Books.

Palombo, S. R. (1980). The cognitive act of dream construction. *Journal of American Academy of Psychoanalysis, 8,* 186–201.

Palombo, S. R. (1987). Can a computer dream? In M. L. Glucksman & S. Warner (Eds.), *Dreams in a new perspective: The royal road revisited* (pp. 59–78). New York: Human Sciences Press.

Perls, F. (1969). *Gestalt therapy verbatim.* New York: Bantam.

Piaget, J. (1962). *Play, dreams, and imitation in childhood.* New York: Norton.

Piaget, J. (1970). Piaget's theory (G. Gellerier & J. Langer, trans). In P. H. Mussen (Ed.), *Carmichael's manual of child psychology* (3rd ed., Vol. 1, pp. 703–732). New York: Wiley.

Piccione, P., Jacobs, G., Kramer, M., & Roth, T. (1977). The relationship between daily activities, emotions, and dream content. *Sleep Research, 6,* 133.

Polster, E., & Polster, M. (1973). *Gestalt therapy integrated.* New York: Random House.

Putnam, F. W. (1989). *Diagnosis and treatment of multiple personality disorder.* New York: Guilford Press.

Rechtschaffen, A., & Buchignani, C. (1983). Visual dimensions and correlates of dream images. *Sleep Research, 12,* 189.

Rechtschaffen, A., Verdone, P., & Wheaton, J. (1963). Reports of mental activity during sleep. *Canadian Psychiatric Association Journal, 8,* 411.

Regan, A. M., & Hill, C. E. (1992). An investigation of what clients and counselors do not say in brief therapy. *Journal of Counseling Psychology, 39,* 168–174.

Reichers, M., Kramer, M., & Trinder, J. (1970). A replication of the Hall–Van de Castle character scale norms. *Psychophysiology, 7,* 238.

Reid, J. R., & Finesinger, J. E. (1952). The role of insight in psychotherapy. *American Journal of Psychiatry, 108,* 726–734.

Reik, T. (1935). *Surprise and the psychoanalyst.* London: Routledge.

Rhodes, R., Hill, C. E., Thompson, B. J., & Elliott, R. (1994). Client retrospective recall of resolved and unresolved misunderstanding events. *Journal of Counseling Psychology, 41,* 473–483.

Robbins, P. R., & Houshi, F. (1983). Some observations on recurrent dreams. *Bulletin of the Menninger Clinic, 47,* 262–265.

Robbins, P. R., & Tanck, R. H. (1992). A comparison of recurrent dreams reported from childhood and recent recurrent dreams. *Imagination, Cognition, and Personality, 11,* 259–262.

Robinson, L. A., Berman, J. S., & Niemeyer, R. A. (1990). Psychotherapy for the treatment of depression: A comprehensive review of controlled outcome research. *Psychological Bulletin, 108,* 30–49.

Rogers, C. R. (1942). *Counseling and psychotherapy.* Boston: Houghton Mifflin.

Rogers, C. R. (1951). *Client-centered therapy: Its current practice, implications, and theory.* Boston: Houghton Mifflin.

Rogers, C. R. (1957). The necessary and sufficient conditions of therapeutic personal change. *Journal of Consulting Psychology, 21,* 93–103.

Roll, S., Hinton, R., & Glazer, M. (1974). Dreams and death: Mexican-Americans vs. Anglo-Americans. *Interamerican Journal of Psychology, 8,* 111–115.

Rosenthal, H. R. (1980). *The discovery of the sub-unconscious in a new approach to dream analysis.* South Miami, FL: Banyan Books.

Ross, R. J., Ball, W. A., Sullivan, K. A., & Caroff, S. N. (1989). Sleep disturbance as the hallmark of posttraumatic stress disorder. *American Journal of Psychiatry, 146,* 697–707.

Rummelhart, D. E., & McClelland, J. L. (Eds.). (1986). *Parallel distributing processing. Explorations in the microstructure of cognition: Vol. I. Foundations.* Cambridge, MA: MIT Press.

Savary, L. M. (1990). Dreams for personal and spiritual growth. In S. Krippner (Ed.), *Dreamtime and dreamwork: Decoding the language of the night* (pp. 6–12). Los Angeles: Tarcher.

Schonbar, R. A. (1968). Confessions of an ex-nondirectivist. In E. F. Hammer (Ed.), *Use of interpretation in treatment: Technique and art* (pp. 55–58). New York: Grune & Stratton.

Schwartz, W. (1990). A psychoanalytic approach to dreamwork. In S. Krippner (Ed.), *Dreamtime and dreamwork: Decoding the language of the night* (pp. 49–58). Los Angeles: Tarcher.

Shuttleworth-Jordan, A. B., & Saayman, G. S. (1989). Differential effects of alternative strategies on psychotherapeutic process in group dream work. *Psychotherapy, 26,* 514–519.

Shuttleworth-Jordan, A. B., Saayman, G. S., & Faber, P. A. (1988). A systematized method for dream analysis in a group setting. *International Journal of Group Psychotherapy, 38,* 473–489.

Silverman, I., & Greer, J. H. (1968). The elimination of a recurrent nightmare by desensitization of a related phobia. *Behaviour Research and Therapy, 6,* 109–111.

Singer, E. (1965). *Key concepts in psychotherapy.* New York: Random House.

Smith, M. L., Glass, G. V., & Miller, T. I. (1980). *The benefits of psychotherapy.* Baltimore: Johns Hopkins University Press.

Snyder, F. (1970). The phenomenology of dreaming. In L. Madow & L. Snow (Eds.), *The psychodynamic implications of the physiological studies on dreams* (pp. 124–151). Springfield, IL: Charles C. Thomas.

Spiegel, S. B., & Hill, C. E. (1989). Guidelines for research on therapist interpretation: Toward greater methodological rigor and relevance to practice. *Journal of Counseling Psychology, 36,* 121–129.

Starker, S. (1973). Aspects of inner experience: Autokinesis, daydreaming, dream recall, and cognitive style. *Perceptual and Motor Skills, 36,* 663–673.

Stein, D. J. (1992). Schemas in the cognitive and clinical sciences: An integrative construct. *Journal of Psychotherapy Integration, 2,* 207–210.

Stiles, W. B., Barkham, M., Shapiro, D. A., & Firth-Cozens, J. (1992). Treatment order and thematic continuity between contrasting psychotherapies: Exploring an implication of the assimilation model. *Psychotherapy Research, 2,* 112–124.

Stiles, W. B., Elliott, R., Llewelyn, S. P., Firth-Cozens, J. A., Margison, F. R., Shapiro, D. A., & Hardy, G. (1990). Assimilation of problematic experiences by clients in psychotherapy. *Psychotherapy, 27,* 411–420.

Stiles, W. B., Meshot, C. M., Anderson, T. M., & Sloan, W. W., Jr. (1992). Assimilation of problematic experiences: The case of John Jones. *Psychotherapy Research, 2,* 81–101.

Strauss, A., & Corbin, J. (1990). *Basics of qualitative research.* Newbury Park, CA: Sage.

Taylor, J. (1983). *Dream work: Techniques for discovering the creative power in dreams.* New York: Paulist Press.

Thompson, B., & Hill, C. E. (1991). Therapist perceptions of client reactions. *Journal of Counseling and Development, 69,* 261–265.

Tonay, V. K. (1993). Personality correlates of dream recall: Who remembers? *Dreaming, 3,* 1–8.

Trenholme, I., Cartwright, R. D., & Greenberg, G. (1984). Dream dimension differences during a life change. *Psychiatry Research, 12,* 35–45.

Trinder, J., & Kramer, M. (1971). Dream recall. *American Journal of Psychiatry, 128,* 296–301.

Ullman, M. (1979). The experiential dream group. In B. B. Wolman (Ed.), *Handbook of dreams* (pp. 407–423). New York: Van Nostrand Reinhold.

Ullman, M. (1987). The dream revisited: Some changed ideas based on a group approach. In M. L. Glucksman & S. L. Warner (Eds.), *Dreams in a new perspective: The royal road revisited* (pp. 119–130). New York: Human Sciences Press.

Ullman, M. (1993). Dreams, the dreamer, and society. In G. Delaney (Ed.), *New directions in dream interpretation* (pp. 41–76). Albany, NY: SUNY Press.

Ullman, M., & Zimmerman, N. (1979). *Working with dreams.* Los Angeles: Tarcher.

Urbina, S. P. (1981). Methodological issues in the quantitative analysis of dream content. *Journal of Personality Assessment, 45,* 71–78.

Van de Castle, R. L. (1994). *The dreaming mind.* New York: Ballantine Books.

Vogel, G. W. (1978). An alternate view of the neurobiology of dreaming. *American Journal of Psychiatry, 135,* 1531–1535.

Vogel, G. W. (1993). Activation-synthesis hypothesis. In M. A. Carskadon (Ed.), *Encyclopedia of sleep and dreaming* (pp. 2–3). New York: Macmillan.

Von Franz, M. L. (1987). *On dreams and death.* Boston: Shambhala.

Von Franz, M. L. (1988). *The way of the dream.* Toronto: Windrose Films.

Von Franz, M. L. (1991). *Dreams.* Boston: Shambhala.

Vossen, A. (1990). Client-centered dream therapy. In G. Lietaer, J. Rombauts, & R. Van Balen (Eds.), *Client-centered and experiential psychotherapy in the nineties.* Leuven, Belgium: Leuven University Press.

Wallach, M. S. (1963). Dream reports and some psychological concomitants. *Journal of Consulting Psychology, 27,* 549.

Warner, S. L. (1983). Can psychoanalytic treatment change dreams? *Journal of the American Academy of Psychoanalysis, 11,* 299–316.

Watson, D. L., & Tharp, R. G. (1989). *Self-directed behavior:Self-modification for personal adjustment.* Pacific Grove, CA: Brooks/Cole.

Webb, D. E., & Fagan, J. (1993). The impact of dream interpretation using psychological kinesiology on the frequency of recurring dreams. *Psychotherapy and Psychosomatics, 59,* 203–208.

Webb, W. B. (1990). Historical perspectives: From Aristotle to Calvin Hall. In S. Krippner (Ed.), *Dreamtime and dreamwork: Decoding the language of the night* (pp. 175–184). Los Angeles: Tarcher.

Webb, W. B. (1993). Dream theories of the ancient world. In M. A. Carskadon (Ed.), *Encyclopedia of sleep and dreaming* (pp. 192–194). New York: Macmillan.

Webb, W. B., & Kersey, J. (1967). Recall of dreams and the probability of stage-1 REM sleep. *Perceptual and Motor Skills, 24,* 627–630.

Weiss, L. (1986). *Dream analysis in psychotherapy.* New York: Pergamon.

Whitman, R., Kramer, M., & Baldridge, B. (1963). Which dream does the patient tell? *Archives of General Psychiatry, 8,* 277–282.

Wilmar, H. A. (1982). Vietnam and madness: Dreams of schizophrenic veterans. *Journal of the American Academy of Psychoanalysis, 10,* 47–65.

Winget, C., Kramer, M., & Whitman, R. (1972). Dreams and demography. *Canadian Psychiatric Association Journal, 17,* 203–208.

Yontef, G., & Simkin, J. S. (1989). Gestalt therapy. In R. Corsini & D. Wedding (Eds.), *Current psychotherapies* (4th ed., pp. 323–362). Itasca, IL: Peacock.

Author Index